SEARCHING FOR CONNECTION

An Exploration of Trauma, Culture, and Hope

SEARCHING FOR
CONNECTION
An Exploration of Trauma, Culture, and Hope

Karen Merriam

TRUTHSAYER
PRESS
San Luis Obispo, California

© 2006 Karen Merriam.
Printed and bound in the United States of America.
All rights reserved. No part of this book may be reproduced or transmitted in any form or by any means, electronic or mechanical, including photocopying, recording, or by an information storage and retrieval system—except by a reviewer who may quote brief passages in a review to be printed in a magazine, newspaper, or on the Internet—without permission in writing from the publisher. For information, please contact Truthsayer Press, P.O. Box 1244, San Luis Obispo, CA 93406.

Although the author and publisher have made every effort to ensure the accuracy and completeness of information contained in this book, we assume no responsibility for errors, inaccuracies, omissions, or any inconsistency herein. Any slighting of people, places, or organizations is unintentional.

COVER: *Inside the Eagle Nebula* used by permission: NOAO/AURA/WIYN
Cover design by Claire Faltesek

Grateful acknowledgment is made to the following
for permission to reprint previously published material:

"Lost" from *Traveling Light: Collected and New Poems*.
Copyright © 1999 by David Wagoner.
Used with permission of the poet and the University of Illinois Press.

"Birdwings" from *The Essential Rumi*. Copyright © 1996 by Coleman Barks, translator.
Used with permission of Coleman Banks.

Excerpts from *A Leg to Stand On* by Oliver Sacks. Copyright © 1985 by Oliver Sacks.
Reprinted with permission of Simon & Schuster Adult Publishing Group.

Excerpts from *Left for Dead* by Beck Weathers. Copyright © 2000 by S. Beck Weathers.
Used by permission of Villard Books, a division of Random House, Inc.

Excerpts from *Wind, Sand and Stars* by Antoine de Saint-Exupéry.
Copyright © 1939 by Antoine de Saint-Exupéry and renewed 1967 by Lewis Galantiére.
Used by permission of Harcourt, Inc.

Excerpts from *Fear No Evil* by Natan Sharansky.
Copyright © 1988 by Random House, Inc. Used by permission of Random House, Inc.

ISBN-13: 978-0-9777334-3-9   ISBN-10: 0-9777334-3-2
LCCN: 2006900027

1st printing 2006

Contents

Acknowledgments vii

1. The Search Begins 3
   A Haunting Memory
   Essential Tools for the Search
      Companion Searchers
      Two-Way Communication
      Confidence
   Looking Ahead

2. Something Is Terribly Wrong 19
   Childbirth Trauma
   An Accident

3. How Connections Are Lost 35
   The Traumatic Process
   Touching the Void
   The Hole in Experience
   Another Kind of Death
   Suicide
   Traumatic Grief

4. Energies to Survive 53
   Creating New Connections
      Words from Afar
      Visions
   The Power of Music
   Hope

5. Principles, Plans, and Strategies 69
Each Struggle Is Unique

6. Legacies: Transmission of Trauma 81
The Power of Silence
A Need to Tell the Story

7. Legacies: The Brain, the Will, and the Body 97
Watch Out for Snipers
When Feelings Have No Words
Cognitive Constriction
Willpower

8. Finding the Face of Compassion 111
Guide, Witness, and Healer
Failures of Compassion
Fear and Fatigue
Attitudes toward Death
The Core of Strength
The Face of All Mankind

9. Pieces Come Together 127
The Beauty of a Rock
Something Is Terribly Wrong
Everyday Signs and Symptoms
Contracts Are Broken
Apocalyptic Visions
The Cultural Imperative for Witnessing

10. Finding Our Connections 145
Transmitting Wisdom
Who We Are
The Rhythms of Hope

Notes 154
References 160
Index 163

Acknowledgments

Without the direct encouragement of Donna Kean, M.S.W., L.C.S.W., most likely this book would not have been written. Donna and the staff and volunteers of Hospice of San Luis Obispo County, CA, have provided me with a continual source of compassionate connection, creative inspiration, and raucous good humor. In my work and in my writing I have endeavored to honor the Hospice commitment to the dignity of human experience.

Steve Silvers, M.F.C.C., stood side-by-side with me to present many of the ideas contained in this book in professional workshops and seminars sponsored by Hospice. His understanding of the concepts related to psychological trauma and his emotional honesty were of inestimable help as I began my search for a way to tell the stories in this book. I extend my sincere thanks also to present and former Hospice staff members, especially Steve Willey and Ingrid Pires, and to Christina, Marilyn, Lidia, Ella, Margaret, Chris, Mary, and Sandy.

Since 1986, the International Society for Traumatic Stress Studies (ISTSS) has served as my professional home. I am deeply grateful to my friends and colleagues at ISTSS for their pioneering research, service, and dedication to sharing their knowledge and practices.

Beverly Engel, M.F.C.C., author, lecturer, psychotherapist, and seminar leader, provided invaluable editorial help and encouragement at important points in the development of the book. Her belief in it has kept me going. Susan Griffin, the gifted feminist writer, poet, essayist, lecturer, teacher, playwright, and filmmaker, helped me to shape and focus the work at a critical juncture. Her insights, guidance, and editorial direction gave me the courage to write more clearly and directly in my own voice.

I offer my deep appreciation and thanks also to my sister, Robin Sharp, and to my dear friends Myra Faust, Jeanie and Andy Greensfelder, Bert Kaplan, Colleen Leigh, Richard Hannibal, and Tracy Haydon for reading the manuscript at various stages and giving me encouragement and support to see the work through to completion. Thanks also to Mary Fullwood, for her many hours of reading and honest critiques.

Finally, to all of the clients I have been fortunate to serve over the past thirty-five years, as well as to the women who volunteered to participate in the pilot research studies I led in the areas of domestic violence and traumatic childbirth, I give sincere thanks for their patience and trust.

Lost

Stand still. The trees ahead and the bushes beside you
    Are not lost. Wherever you are is called Here,
    And you must treat it as a powerful stranger,
    Must ask permission to know it and be known.
    The forest breathes. Listen. It answers,
    I have made this place around you.
If you leave it, you may come back again, saying Here.
    No two trees are the same to Raven.
    No two branches are the same to Wren.
    If what a tree or a bush does is lost on you,
You are surely lost. Stand still. The forest knows
    Where you are. You must let it find you.

        —DAVID WAGONER

CHAPTER 1

The Search Begins

"...that others may live."
—NASAR

The shrill warning tone of my Search and Rescue pager startled me as I was preparing dinner one winter evening eight years ago. I could barely make out the words of the voice message that followed, strangled as they were by static: "Call Out...Missing...Eighty-four year-old..." The crackling noise took over, obscuring the rest of the message. I looked longingly at my warm food on the stove, then moved to the phone to dial the Search and Rescue (SAR) dispatcher to learn the details of the search being organized.

Because I served as a volunteer employee of the County Sheriff's Department, on the SAR K-9 team, I had the option to say "no" to a call out for any reason: "My dog is tired; I'm hungry; I've been on too many searches lately; there's a movie I want to see." But this was the call we trained for, a priority call that required immediate response without weighing preferences. It would be dark in less than an hour, bringing deep cold with the night, and an elderly person was missing.

Automatically, I changed into my uniform as I listened to the dispatcher on the phone. A widowed, white, male, age eighty-four, wearing tan cotton pants, white polo shirt, and sneakers, was missing from an athletic club where he had been waiting for his son to finish his workout. He failed to meet his son at their car as planned. He had not been seen for over an hour. He was known to be "confused"; however, he had no prior history of wandering off. His name was William.

I would wait until I was on scene to learn more information about William. Now I needed to get all my gear together, as well as my dog's, and get there as quickly as possible. Even on the central coast of California it can be cold enough on a February night to kill an old man who has wandered off in only thin slacks and a cotton shirt.

The club is located in a rural residential area just fifteen minutes from where I lived. It is surrounded by woods, orchards, and new housing tracts, each competing for a little space in a narrow valley, and it is bordered on the south by a swift creek. When I got there thirty minutes after the call, several sheriff's deputies were at the parking lot staging area. Only one other SAR member, Denny, had arrived so far. He was a relatively new person in the Unit, as was I, and he was not a part of the specialized K-9 team.

Checklists of procedures scrolled through my mind as I outfitted my dog, Babe, with her Search Dog vest, her harness, her thirty-foot lead, and a neon-yellow chemical light stick to make it easier to follow her in the dark. I put on my own layers of clothing and my heavy boots, and then loaded my pack with first-aid supplies, four liters of water for Babe and for me, power bars and kibble treats, a compass, a whistle, and fully ten pounds of additional miscellaneous gear that I might or might not need.

The deputy-in-charge came over to ask if I was willing to start searching right away. Absolutely, I said. Time was critical, and I had the most valuable search tool needed in this kind of incident: a tracking dog. Babe was, in fact, the only Search and Rescue tracking dog with statewide certification for hundreds of miles around. Never mind that some people made fun of her because she was an unusual breed to take on such a big job. Like most English cocker spaniels, she stands no more than shin high. She has the head and face of a springer spaniel—with long nose and even

CHAPTER 1: THE SEARCH BEGINS

longer ears—and the short legs and trim body of the smaller American cocker spaniel. Her mostly white coat, marked with black spots, and her black ears and eye patches cause children to think that she might be one of the 101 Dalmatians of movie fame.

The deputy briefed me with the little information available. William had last been seen by a security guard at the gate to the club who said "he thought he saw" the old man walking out toward the road, but he couldn't be sure. The son reported that his father was in fairly good health and that he walked slowly, with a shuffle. This was welcome news. At least we had a PLS—Place Last Seen—to start from, and our missing man might not have been able to wander too far.

Now I needed to gather a "scent article," some item with William's specific scent on it, so that Babe could follow his direction of travel. The deputy took me to the son's car and indicated that William had sat in the passenger's seat just a few hours ago on his way to the club. Unfortunately, there were no items of his clothing or other personal belongings available that we could bag and take with us as scent articles. However, when we were ready to go, I would direct Babe to sniff the car seat area, give her the commands to "Track! Find William!" and hope there would be enough of his specific scent to enable her do her job.

Denny agreed to team up with Babe and me. It is a firm rule in SAR that no one searches alone, only in teams. Since handheld radios were in short supply in the Unit, I would have to depend on Denny's radio to communicate with the deputies, and with the incident commander when the rest of the SAR members arrived and set up a base of operations. I had a flashlight, but Denny had forgotten to bring his. He also had forgotten to bring water. Not a good sign. One radio, one flashlight, two inexperienced searchers: this was beginning to feel a bit precarious.

It's hard to distinguish excitement from anxiety at a time like this. There is ample adrenaline activated to fuel both. Babe was watching me carefully, eager to start the search. Once she has her vest on, she knows she is at work. The words "search" and "track" have specific meanings for her. They tell her the kind of job to be done and how to do it. She knows by these words that she is looking for a living human being and that she is to detect, match, and then follow the path of the millions of scattered skin cells that the missing person has sloughed off in his normal movements as we all do.

We were finally ready. I asked Denny to walk behind me and watch for clues that William may have left along the ground or in the brush. I would be busy watching Babe's every move: every turn of her head, stiffening of her back, shift of her ears, direction of her tail. Babe and I understood each other's language of signs and sounds. The success of our search would depend on our deeply developed interconnection of language, skill, intuition, willingness, and trust.

And so we began the search, first at the car where Babe took William's scent, then at the security gate, the PLS. While I held my end of her thirty-foot lead, Babe ranged in a wide arc, looking for the scent trail, casting about for the strongest possibilities. This time of waiting and watching the tracking dog begin her work is hard. It highlights one's dependence on her skill and her decisions. Only Babe could know with certainty whether William had come this way and where he was going.

Suddenly, she pulled strongly, decidedly, on the lead, taking a direction straight away from the club toward the road. Even on asphalt pavement a tracking dog can find and follow an individual's specific scent trail. We were at a trot now. I urged Denny to run ahead and stop any cars that might be coming along the curving rural road in the dusk. I wanted to maintain our trajectory without interruption.

Babe was so certain of her course. After traveling several hundred yards from the security gate, she crossed the two-lane road, then took a sharp right turn to travel along the gravel verge for five hundred feet or more. Then, all at once, she veered left, turning away from the road at a ninety-degree angle, and headed into the woods. I could hear the creek close at hand now on our right. Abruptly, the lead went slack, and we

CHAPTER 1: THE SEARCH BEGINS

stopped. A large gate, almost five feet tall and ten feet wide blocked our way. A padlock secured it shut. Babe sniffed its horizontal metal bars, traveled its width, and jumped up to catch the scent on rungs above her head. She was ready to go forward, to squeeze through or under the rails. Denny and I could climb over easily.

Now that we were stopped, now that our forward thrust was halted, we could take a moment to evaluate our plan and call back to the deputies to tell them where we were and where we were headed. I had never been through this gate before, and I didn't know where the path led. Was it private land? Would we need permission to go further? It was dark now, and I could see only a few feet of the gravel trail beyond the gate. Could William have climbed this gate?

Denny took out the radio and pushed the key to talk. Nothing. No squawk, no tone, nothing. He adjusted every knob, turned the power on and off. Nothing. The radio was dead. Without a working radio we couldn't go forward. That was another basic rule. Going it alone and going without the ability to communicate with base were not options on a search. Denny agreed to run back to the parking lot to get another radio. He took my flashlight with him for his safety since it was now very dark.

As I waited, I got a sense of how cold this night would become. I was eager to get moving again, to encourage Babe to follow the scent trail, worried that she might forget who we were looking for. Small bits of doubt found a foothold in this opening of time. Perhaps Babe was wrong. Perhaps the subject hadn't come this way. Surely he couldn't have climbed this gate. And do I know enough to be the lead team in this search? We waited. Denny didn't return.

We had to go back. We couldn't continue the search for William. Unable to explain to Babe my reasons, the rules we had to follow, I could only apologize and tug on her lead to turn her. We walked slowly, Babe now at my side, the quarter mile or so back to the staging area. By now other SAR members were arriving, including the leader of the K-9 team with her German shepherd. Because she was the more experienced searcher, with a well-seasoned area-search dog, she was assigned to pick up the search where Babe and I had left off. We had found the direction of travel; they would continue the search.

After getting a new radio and a new teammate, I was assigned to check out a different area around the clubhouse. Search and Rescue can be a bit like the military: once given an order, one is expected to follow it. But I knew that William was somewhere in the woods on the other side of that gate.

As soon as I completed my assignment by the clubhouse, my teammate and I headed back across the road with Babe, and I gave Babe the command again: "Track! Find William!" We climbed the gate and headed into the dark with Babe thirty feet in the lead pulling strongly. She had not forgotten. The woods were thick on both sides of a narrow path, creating a quiet even in the midst of the activity of the search. I was excited, and Babe was working well. To see the extraordinary talent of the tracking dog at work is a thrilling experience. She can and will ignore all other scents, even of critters and of food that normally she adores, and follow only that scent of the person for whom she is asked to look. We moved forward steadily for about a half mile.

The radio I was carrying suddenly broke the silence. "The subject is found!" The voice sounded pleased and relieved. Now I could see a dim light through the trees just ahead.

We broke into a small clearing several feet to the left of the trail, and I saw him: I saw William sitting on a tree stump in the darkness, the light of a flashlight illuminating his face and torso. He looked bewildered. Babe ran over to him, touching her nose to his leg. She had found the right person after all—she had done her job. I praised her and then rewarded her with food treats. We were not the first to reach him, but we had found William.

Soon more searchers arrived with lights and radios and questions for William, none of which he could answer. He didn't know where he was, how he had come to be there, or what was happening around him. He felt

CHAPTER 1: THE SEARCH BEGINS

fine, he said. He wasn't injured nor had the cold affected him yet. He was tired, he said. In a little while, he accepted help to walk back down the path to his waiting son.

I stayed on for a few moments in the clearing after William left with the other searchers. What a lonely place it was when everyone had gone. The air was still and damp; darkness filled the space.

A Haunting Memory

Why does the image of William, alone in the clearing, continue to haunt me? Of all the searches I took part in during my six years of work with Search and Rescue, why do I remember this one with such persistence and in such detail? Not all of our searches ended so successfully. There were times we were not able to find the missing person. For instance: the sheriff's deputy who went hiking and never came back; the paraglider who sailed into the air over the ocean and was never seen again. Other times we found a body: the child who had drowned; the man who had been murdered.

Yet, even now, eight years later, I see clearly—in my mind's eye—William, sitting alone on the tree stump in the clearing in the woods: a man utterly alone. I see how it was for him before the searchers came, before Babe touched him with her nose. It was dark and cold, and he was alone and confused and lost, without connection to anything he understood within or around him. Was this an experience that we would call trauma? It's not really possible to say, since William himself could not describe what he felt or what meaning the moment had for him. Each person must define traumatic experience for him- or herself. It is a deeply subjective assessment.

It is possible, however, in witnessing another's wounds to find a likeness of one's own experience that is buried deep in memory. I believe the picture of William alone in the clearing remains so vivid for me because his aloneness is deeply a part of my own experience. In the illumination of his presence in the darkness of the clearing, I saw a reflection of myself—of my own experience of utter aloneness—at a time long before I had words to record it in the memory of language. Yet, it is bedrock. I know that, like William, I waited in the dark, bewildered and lost: waited for someone to find me and take me to safety. There is no event in my memory to which I can attach this ancient awareness, no time, no place—only a memory of the feelings.

Is this a memory of trauma? I am certain that it is an experience that has echoed throughout my life and has given form and direction to who I am and what I do. It has left me with a legacy of fear, a terror of becoming lost that cannot be assuaged by reason, skill, or maturity. It has impelled me to understand its cause, to offer others comfort, as I search for my own, and to find a path out of that place of terrible darkness. I have been both the missing subject and the searcher, looking for the connections within myself and to the world that will ensure my safety and survival.

Essential Tools for the Search

Other memories of the search for William have also remained unsettling to me over the years. Even though we found our subject, I came away from the experience with an awareness that I had been missing some essential tools I needed to do the work.

First, I had begun the search without waiting for the arrival of the rest of the SAR teams from the Unit, reliable companions who could aid and support my work. Second, I lacked an essential means of communication, the two-way radio. Without the ability to communicate with others and to my base, I had the potential for becoming lost also. Third, I did not have a teammate I could trust. And fourth, I lacked total confidence in myself and in my dog Babe. For long moments during the search I doubted both of us. In short, when I started out on the search for William, there were important ways in which I was not ready.

CHAPTER 1: THE SEARCH BEGINS

And there is something else here that needs to be explored: something that speaks to larger, internal emotional issues, not just external readiness. I have set out many times before to explore the face of trauma, only to turn back. And even when I have found the subject, as we found William, I have been left with the sense of something missing, of work left undone, of understanding left incomplete. Only now do I feel ready to put into place all the pieces, the fragments of understanding I've accumulated over the years, to gain a more complete picture of traumatic experience—my own and others'—and of the ways in which individual experiences of trauma may be reflected in our collective life and expressed in our culture.

To see the work of this search through to completion, I have on hand certain basic tools: my computer; my years of study of literature, psychology, and social systems; my love of language; my clinical experience as a social worker and psychotherapist for over thirty years; and my enjoyment of adventure and exploration. But more than these, I now have with me also the key elements I lacked in my search for William. As I describe below, to undertake this book, which is an exploration and expression of the experience and meaning of trauma, I have brought together a team to serve as companions-in-search, to give me a solid base, and I have been able to identify a special kind of two-way communication that gives depth and purpose to my efforts. And, finally, I have gained the confidence needed to see this search through to its conclusion.

Companion Searchers

In my personal and professional search to understand traumatic experience and its aftermath, I have been fortunate to find many others who share my deep interest and passion. I think of them now as my reliable search companions, who encourage and inform me all along the way. They form my base of operations.

I should explain, however, that, although I find myself in dialogue with them often, most of these fellow searchers I speak of do not know me. They are writers, poets, composers, physicians, and artists who, by their works, profess that they, also, have been or still are searchers who wish to understand and express the nature of traumatic experience. All are witnesses. They speak with the special words, music, and honest representation that traumatic experience engenders. Their particular contributions to my work will become readily apparent and explicit as we go forward in these pages. For now, I offer a few brief introductions to illustrate the importance of these companions-in-search to me and to understanding trauma.

One of my earliest and continuing mentors is Robert Jay Lifton, a psychiatrist, researcher, and writer of international renown. I began reading his work on brainwashing and other experiences of prisoners of war when I was in my teens. Only in hindsight can I understand that even then I was looking for clues to understand certain emotional experiences in my own life that seemed to have no outward, objective correlates.

Throughout the years Lifton's analyses of the people who have been part of traumatic events have influenced and expanded my thinking. Most recently, his exploration of cults and apocalyptic visionaries in *Destroying the World to Save It: Aum Shinrikyō, Apocalyptic Violence, and the New Global Terrorism* provides a cautionary study of terror, martyrdom, and global threat in the 21st century. Reading Lifton, I have gained the courage to look into the abyss of suffering, no matter how painful or full of dread, and to record and bear witness to what I see.

Elie Wiesel, a Nobel Laureate for Peace, journalist, author, and public speaker, has given counsel to all who will listen not to forget those who died and those who survived the Holocaust of the Second World War. We must not be silent, he exhorts, though we tell the stories of those who have been silenced. We must not abandon responsibility for those who are voiceless because of war, because of suffering, because of evil, because of

CHAPTER 1: THE SEARCH BEGINS

traumatic experience. Wiesel is that companion who grabs one by the arm and says: we cannot forget where we have been if we hope to move forward out of the darkness of the past. I have been both shaken and emboldened by his words.

In an early autobiographical book, *A Leg to Stand On*, Oliver Sacks, the neurologist and well-known popular writer provides an account of an injury he sustained while hiking alone in the mountains in Norway and his subsequent hospitalization. It is a compelling narration of the traumatic process. Throughout his many books and articles, Sacks asserts that who we are is defined not only by a name, an occupation, a belief, or a set of emotions, but that we find definition also in our relationship to our bodies. The integrity of the whole person is dependent on the relations between all of the parts of what we call the self. If the body is damaged, the soul may suffer also. Indeed, both science and common sense tell us that terrible fear and pain may be recorded deeply within the structure and functions of the body.

What draws me to Sacks is his passion and honesty. He is not afraid to speak of the terror and madness that are part of the traumatic process, even when it means talking about the most personal aspects of his own experience of traumatic injury and healing.

Terry Tempest Williams, first with her book *Refuge* and then with her many books and essays that have followed, has also become a trusted companion in my exploration of the topography of traumatic experience. A women of deep spiritual awareness and candor, she writes forcefully about loss—loss of self, loss of a beloved—in the context of the losses we face every day in the larger natural environment. I take strength from her determination to look straight into the dark dread of extinction—both personal and collective, as well as in the natural world around us—and to report what she sees.

Joe Simpson sustained terrible wounds, both physical and psychological, in the course of his many mountaineering achievements. His books, among them *Touching the Void*—from which a documentary film has recently been made—and *This Game of Ghosts*, have taken me into a world that I might never have known without his help. The metaphor of trauma as a dark abyss takes on new meaning as Simpson describes his experience of lying stranded, deep in a crevasse on Siula Grande in the remote Peruvian Andes. Both Simpson and Ruth Anne Kocour, also a mountaineer, who has written *Facing the Extreme*, remind me with their stories of survival that it's not possible to know what strengths one has until one is driven by the deepest desperation and desire to live to struggle to the end of one's endurance. They attest, also, to the terrible toll such experiences of trauma take on a person. They remind me that one doesn't "get over" trauma: one bears it for a lifetime, finding ways—or not—to integrate the experience into one's life.

Maya Angelou, the dancer, writer, teacher, and poet; Antoine de Saint-Exupéry, the pilot and author of *The Little Prince* and *Wind, Sand, and Stars*, and Bernard Lown, the Nobel Peace Laureate, pioneering cardiologist, and author of *The Lost Art of Healing*, are also among the many eloquent and generous people who have assisted me in my search. Their unique experiences and understandings of trauma inform my thought, my methods of investigation, and the language I choose to talk about trauma. They have helped me to explore how traumatic experience begins, what it looks and feels like from deep within, and how life evolves in its aftermath. Without them, surely I would have turned back from this exploration; for to understand trauma is too difficult and complex a task to undertake alone, without the sure help of wise companions who provide a steady base of support.

Two-Way Communication

One doesn't need a two-way radio to write a book, in the way it was a necessary tool in Search and Rescue. Yet there is a kind of reciprocal communication, a deep certainty of connection with one's companions-in-search, that makes bearable the solitary activity of looking into the face

CHAPTER 1: THE SEARCH BEGINS

of personal and collective experiences of profound trauma. Natan Sharansky has described just such a kind of reciprocal communication in his book *Fear No Evil*.

From 1977 to 1986 Sharansky was held captive in Soviet prisons as a political prisoner. In the lonely days and years of his confinement, he developed a certainty that an "interconnection of human souls" exists, one that transcends the limitations of space and time. This sense of sure connection extended not just to his family and fellow prisoners in far-off cells but even to the great characters of literature, such as Hamlet and Ulysses. As he recalled them and their stories, he felt that their "struggles reverberated with my own, their laughter with mine." Their presence reached in to him through the prison bars, giving him strength and dispelling his utter aloneness.

In what Sharansky describes as a "curious" awareness that emerged as he spent time remembering the words and actions of these characters from literature, he understood his own importance to them. He felt his importance to those characters who had also endured great hardship and grief and had struggled to maintain their integrity in the face of overwhelming dangers, just as he was attempting to do. In this "reverse connection," he felt that "not only was it important to me how these characters behaved in various circumstances, but it was also important to them, who had been created many centuries ago, to know how I was acting today."

In this reciprocity of living people with ancestors, with characters from stories who shared his struggles, and with those not yet created, Sharansky believes there is an implicit responsibility: an obligation to make decisions that honor not only his own life but their lives also.

Although I have relied on my companions from literature and art, medicine and mountaineering to inform my understanding of trauma, I have also needed the touch, the voices, and the company of trusted friends to keep me anchored while I have explored the dark places of suffering and loss. They have provided an essential safety without which I could not have proceeded.

Confidence

There's a kind of confidence that is borne of bravado. Many of the young men and women new to Search and Rescue provided shining examples of this kind of false assurance of skill. Their bluster reminded me of the solitary game of lost and found I often played when I was about sixteen years old. I would drive out into the countryside on unfamiliar roads to see if I could get lost. With relief and reassurance, I always found my way home. I didn't understand then that I was truly afraid of being lost.

In any search to understand traumatic experience, one will always get lost. Real confidence is needed: a kind of trust in one's intuition, in one's deep instinct and ability to withstand the impact of the results of the search and to come home to oneself when the search is over. On searches for SAR, my dog Babe was a visible representation of instinct. She could *see* what was not visible to me; she could scent, or sense, the direction of the subject's travel; she could tell me when the person had wandered off the path; she could circumvent difficult obstacles; she could "make the find"; and she always knew the way back to base.

Gretel Ehrlich, the well-known nature writer, writes about the special role her two dogs played in her struggle to survive a direct hit by lightning. "Harnessed dogs," Ehrlich explains, have long been regarded as one of the "supernatural helpers" whose work it is to "carry the human spirit forward."

Babe was, and continues to be, my helper and my guide; she reminds me of the need to trust my instinct, and—by her example—to sense the invisible signs and clues that take me to the subject, to an understanding of traumatic loss, others' and my own. Without trust in my guide and in myself, joined with the other tools essential to the search, I could not have completed the mission of this book.

CHAPTER 1: THE SEARCH BEGINS

Looking Ahead

It has taken me most of a lifetime to ready myself to stand at this intersection where the stories of experiences and aftereffects of trauma that I have heard and have witnessed meet the story that I have lived. At this junction the work of the book begins: to bring together the experiences, both personal and received from others, to form a unified understanding of trauma and its legacy.

With intuition in the lead, I have set out from this starting place to explore the first sign of trauma: an awareness that "something is terribly wrong." This sense of terrible dread and foreboding signals that an experience—which may have begun as ordinary—has become one with potential for great harm.

Next I explore what is meant by the word "trauma," what events produce traumatic experience, and how to determine when trauma has occurred. Although the meaning of the word may at first seem obvious, in fact, trauma is not easy to define. It is both a process and a state of being. It is an experience of everything and nothing at once. It defies words, yet demands expression, over and over.

When confronted with stories of terrible suffering, I have uttered the words I know are spoken by many: how can anyone survive such terrible wounds? Of course, there are as many explanations of survival as there are accounts of the circumstances of the traumatic injuries themselves. In this book I have searched to understand not only what has helped individuals to endure traumatic experience but also what diverse efforts to survive have in common that can serve as guides for us all.

The legacy of traumatic experience is long and wide and deep. Out of the terrible fragmentation and chaos of the losses engendered by trauma, new connections must be forged. Otherwise trauma takes a terrible toll, affecting not just families but the larger society. Many questions arise: How does wholeness become possible? How is trauma passed from one generation to another? What of those who find no resolution to their wounds? I have taken time to explore these and related questions carefully.

The essential role of witnesses to traumatic suffering, both our own and others, leads naturally into a deeper discussion of how it is possible to provide support and empathic understanding to those who have experienced profound trauma. One does not always choose to be a helper or to lend a willing hand; yet it is clear that compassion itself, reaching into the heart of traumatic suffering to provide a vital connection to another, is transformative.

Finally, the path of understanding we have been following brings us to a new intersection. We arrive at a place where personal and collective human stories of trauma intersect with the sensual, natural world, in which cell and rock, wind and anemone, hawk and blade of grass speak to us. It is almost certain, I believe, that if we listen deeply and openly, we will see and we will know that something is terribly wrong. Understanding our own human traumatic experience must lead to a deeper understanding of the enormity of the environmental trauma that is taking place, in which untold numbers of species are becoming extinct every day and the very life of our planet is threatened. Violence and woundedness echo across and within the oceans. Once fertile plains and lakes filled with fresh water have become wastelands.

These are our losses. The interconnection of human souls is only a small part of the larger interdependence of all things, animate and inanimate, in our universe. Each day we encounter new evidence that we are in danger. Something is terribly wrong. We must be brave enough to say these words aloud. The healing of our human lives depends on the health of all life.

CHAPTER 2

Something Is Terribly Wrong

"...something is terribly missing, some essential ingredient has been neglected, some necessary aspect of life has been dangerously overlooked, set aside, or simply forgotten..."
—DAVID ABRAM

Warnings of danger often come to us from the outside world: in the form of a siren, a train whistle at a crossing, or a car horn honking at an intersection. Such warnings may also be heard in the voice of a worried parent: "Watch Out! Be Careful!" They are intended to affect behavior: to urge a person to move, to take action, to do what's necessary to survive.

Warnings of danger may also be sounded from inside a person's awareness. As I have listened to and read countless stories of traumatic suffering and survival, I have been struck by how many people have used the same phrase—"something is terribly wrong"—to express an internal awareness of grave and imminent danger that precedes a downward spiral into trauma. Often the perception of danger is accompanied by the thought, "I am going to die." This internal experience is not just worry, not just anxiety but both of these and much more: it also includes a feeling of dread and of terrible foreboding. It is the expression of the body, the mind, the emotions, and the spirit of a person all at once, in one concerted voice of alarm.

The perception that something is terribly wrong often signals the start of the process of traumatic experience. If immediate intervention does not take place, the experience of trauma proceeds. By this I mean that the sure connections that protect and maintain the integrity and the wholeness of the person begin to pull apart and to disintegrate as the experience of trauma deepens. The vital connections—to oneself and to others—are lost, so that the individual becomes utterly alone, abandoned in the experience of trauma, whether on a mountain, in a prison cell, in a hospital room, in the rubble of an earthquake, or in the wake of abuse.

A person may have an awareness that something is terribly wrong but have no opportunity to take action or to summon help. The greater the delay in receiving an intervention by others or from inner resources, the more catastrophic the consequences, including death. Often, however, there are opportunities early on in the traumatic process in which fragile connections within the parts of the self, and of the self to others, can be supported in order to change the experience so that the basic strengths and integrity of the person are maintained and traumatic disintegration is prevented. We have learned this lesson in the field of emergency medicine: early response saves lives. But we have yet to understand that the same principles can be applied to psychological emergencies.

For this reason it is important to look closely at those first crucial moments of an experience, in which the threat of terrible danger and injury is perceived, to understand what opportunities might exist to prevent its dangerous progress. My work with a research project on trauma in childbirth underscored for me this important lesson.

Childbirth Trauma

In the early 1990s, in Seattle, Washington, I gathered together a team of investigators to design and conduct a preliminary research study to explore and understand more fully women's experiences of trauma in

CHAPTER 2: SOMETHING IS TERRIBLY WRONG

giving birth. Transcribed words of women who participated in the study provide moving examples of the process of traumatic experience as it unfolds, starting with the women's perception that something was going terribly wrong.

Our team initiated the research study in response to a growing awareness among some clinicians in the fields of psychology, nursing, social work, and midwifery that there is a peculiar silence that surrounds the more difficult, sometimes overwhelming experiences that women endure during childbirth. The silence arises from assumptions that are pervasive in American culture. First, according to both popular and professional opinion, because childbirth is a "normal" activity, one expected of women, it cannot, by definition, be considered a traumatic experience. A second, companion assumption is one that describes pain as an inevitable part of childbirth, which must be endured without complaint or consequence, regardless of its magnitude. Accordingly, when a woman speaks of foreboding, of terror, of being overwhelmed, or of a sense of terrible loss and sadness in association with her birthing experience, such expressions are often interpreted as indications of the woman's failure in her role as child bearer and of psychological pathology.

Our goal, as a research team, was to learn from each woman in the study about her experience through her own words (as opposed to providing a checklist or a set of questions based on other people's words and assumptions). We were determined to listen to and record faithfully each woman's description. In doing so, we hoped to collect ethnographic data about traumatic childbirth that would increase our understanding. We also offered empathic connection by listening deeply to what each woman told us and by the very fact of wanting to hear her story fully. We agreed that the women's words would tell us all that we needed to know. Each interview lasted a minimum of two hours.

In order to determine who would be selected to be interviewed, women who had volunteered to talk about their childbirth experiences were asked a simple question: "Would you consider that you have experienced trauma in giving birth?" Since one of the main purposes of the study was to learn how each woman defines the experience for herself, the word "trauma" was not discussed or given a definition. This posed no challenge to the women who responded: each knew exactly what her own definition of trauma was, and she stated without equivocation that her experience was—or was not—traumatic.

Two separate groups emerged easily and clearly: women whose birthing experience may have entailed pain and difficulties but on the whole was seen as manageable, tolerable, and generally positive and women who were overwhelmed, who descended into a chasm of pain, terror, timelessness, and utter aloneness—and for whom the traumatic memory persisted long after the event. From the many women who volunteered to participate in the study, two groups of about equal size formed. That so many women defined their childbirth experiences as traumatic was a new and disturbing finding in and of itself.

What follows is a composite of some of the voices of the women who described their childbirth experiences as traumatic. When combined, these selections from the transcribed interviews of their narrative accounts offer an accurate description of certain important aspects of trauma that was described by all.

The first selections speak of the descent into the traumatic experience.

— *My pain was beyond any comprehension. It was so intense, I thought I was going to die....No matter how I tried to breathe or calm my body down, the pain...it was just...I wanted to die.*

— *I told my husband that something was wrong....The character of the contractions had changed. I was not able to handle them with breathing, and I couldn't understand it, and no one was talking to me....I was screaming*

CHAPTER 2: SOMETHING IS TERRIBLY WRONG

in pain with these contractions. I was begging people to cut the Pitocin off, that I didn't need it any more. There's something wrong!

— I knew they were doing things around me, but I couldn't understand why nobody would talk to me. Nobody would answer me. Nobody would touch me. Nobody came up and held my hand and talked to me...

— My perceptions that I was, in fact, pregnant were totally lost for a period of minutes....And then I was in the delivery room, and I was frantically pushing, and they kept yelling at me to push, to push, to push, and I kept saying, "I'm trying, I'm trying."...I was exhausted, and...[the baby's] shoulder got stuck....They lost her pulse. They had to unwrap the cord from around her neck. I was in constant, constant agony.

(This baby was finally born, by surgical intervention, under anaesthesia, after 72 hours of labor.)

— I couldn't even process that I had this baby. I couldn't even hold her for a little while. It was so bizarre. All of a sudden, pulling myself back to the point of remembering...and here was this baby, and she was all right, and finally I could hold her. And I started gluing my perceptions back in place, but it was very distorted for a while.

— To me it was a real humiliating experience....The labor was unbearable for me, and I kept saying, "I can't take it." And everyone around me kept saying, "Yes, you can," and invalidating my feelings and my experience. My husband said he left the room twice to cry...and the second time he went and found the doctor and said, "You've got to do something!"

— The physical pain of my birth experience was—it just felt like I wasn't there. There's this big thing that was a deep—sort of like in the bottom of a well being tortured.

SEARCHING FOR CONNECTION

This next selection speaks of the desire to understand why this overwhelming experience could not be coped with psychologically and to find meaning in the traumatic experience.

— *You feel powerless. I think that you can become a victim of trauma when you have no power in your situation or no control....I realize that the whole experience of being pregnant and having a baby is somewhat beyond your control. You really have to give over to the grace of life. That's what I felt like I had to do.*

— *But a woman needs to be able to say what she needs when she's in that moment. That's the kind of control I'm talking about. And I think you can experience trauma when people say to you, "Those things aren't important; you're not going to get them; you can't have them." And they just take your decision-making power away.*

— *The thing I found in the hospital more than anything is that the needs of the mother are not considered important. It's the needs of the baby. And they don't see that the needs of the mother can be complementary and unified, really, one dependent on the other, interdependent. What I felt was: What I need is what my son needs. I need to be with him, and he needs to be with me. And they said, "No, he needs medicine in a bottle. You need rest, away from each other."*

— *I was looked at as someone who was kind of an emotional basket case. I called myself that because that's how I felt I was looked at. But when I look back on it now, I think about [how] all those tears and all that anger and sadness and confusion was so justified and normal. But I was treated as if I was like a mental case. There's like a lack of connection there: the intense spiritual and emotional significance of a birth is not—was not considered in my case.*

CHAPTER 2: SOMETHING IS TERRIBLY WRONG

— *I realized there were things about her birth I couldn't put in perspective, I couldn't put in order, and I didn't understand—that there were these huge holes.*

Many women had flashbacks, reliving the traumatic experience.

— *I kept having these crying periods and, worse than anything, shortly after I left the hospital...I would have these flashbacks. I would have periods where...I would be feeling the same pain that I went through when I was in labor with her. I'd be feeling the same pain I went through when I delivered her. I would feel the same frustration that I felt right after I had her when I was trying to put my head back together.*

And often, grief continued for many years.

— *I still have a sensation of grief, of massive grief....I have awful nightmares. I wake up in these drenching cold sweats.*

Above all, women continued to look for wholeness they had lost.

— *I don't think I'm over her birth. I think there's some parts that are patched okay, but I think that there's a lot of emotional scars left with it. The whole thing around caregivers and people who just assume: "Well, we're just going to cut you open and da, de, da, de, da." Just to assume these things and to put the spiritual or the emotional side apart kind of like they're cataloging you. They want to take you as a physical entity. It really, really still bothers me a whole lot.*

As illustrated in these excerpts, for some women who described their experiences as being traumatic, early in the birthing process there was a certainty that "something is wrong." From that point forward, dread became the primary emotional component. It announced the fact that a serious problem was at hand, bringing danger to both mother and baby. Whether the problem that the mother perceived was physical, such as the baby's shoulder being stuck in the birth canal, or emotional, such as the depletion of her confidence, the danger was real and imminent.

Often, however, her perceptions were not understood or validated by the attending medical personnel or others giving supportive care.

As the birth continued, the women described a sense of mounting danger and dread, moving from the turbulence of confusion, pain, and activity toward the silence of the eye of a storm. In that silent center of traumatic experience, their narratives suggest, time lost its meaning; the presence of supportive (or non-supportive) people around the woman faded; the notion of help slipped away; and the sense of aloneness became complete. Then, as the trajectory of the storm swept the silence away, the crash of activity began again, leaving the woman bewildered, defenseless, and voiceless. Her own experience had no words, and her efforts to get help could not be heard or understood by those around her. As a final injury, these deeply traumatized women were often labeled and treated by those attending them as "whiners," "uncooperative," and "hysterical."

It becomes clear from this composite of voices that the early sense of invalidation of the woman's self-knowledge and perception of her circumstances sets the tone for all that is to come. The mother's relationship with and awareness of the needs of her own changing body and of her growing baby gained during the months of the pregnancy often are not given credence in the urgent moments of the birth. Ideas of what is "supposed to happen" come into conflict with the mother's own understanding of what is occurring within her body and to the life of her fragile baby. At this critical time, it is of vital importance to listen to the insights of the mother.

The invalidation of perception and needs expressed by the women in their childbirth experiences was a key component of the ongoing process of trauma. It began early and continued long after the birth was complete.

CHAPTER 2: SOMETHING IS TERRIBLY WRONG

In our sample, the births described had taken place from two years to twenty years prior to the interview. For some of the women, the research interview provided the first opportunity to tell their story in full detail and to have it listened to completely, seriously, and with respect. For some, it was the first time that they felt they had an opportunity to think of themselves not as "whiners" or as "a basket case" but to acknowledge that their experiences had meaning and significance, not just for them but for others also. They saw their contributions to the research study as a way to help other women.

The stories that were related as a part of the research study were echoed again and again by other women who, unsolicited, confirmed with their own stories what we learned in the study. Whether I was sitting with a painting group in the high plains of New Mexico or talking with a neighbor, once I mentioned my work and interest in this subject, narratives of traumatic births came pouring out. This proved true for the others on the research team also.

For instance, a friend named Sally, who is a nurse and whose husband is a doctor, told me of her terrifying experience with the birth of their first child. Immediately after the birth, Sally said, she was essentially abandoned while all attention was focused on the baby, who had some minor difficulties. Because she was a nurse, Sally noticed symptoms of something going terribly wrong within her body. She was bleeding profusely, yet no one seemed concerned or attended to her. After many efforts to get help from the medical staff, she finally gave up and lost confidence in her own perceptions that she was in danger. While her dread mounted, her hope faded.

Some short time later, when her husband arrived on the scene and saw what was happening to Sally, he intervened, though it was against "protocol." He declared his wife's situation an emergency and summoned medical staff to help her. Once the staff members gave their attention to Sally, it was acknowledged that she was bleeding-out and would soon die if immediate measures weren't taken. She was rushed to surgery. It is likely that if Sally had been listened to when she first expressed that something was wrong, the trauma of her near-death experience could have been avoided.

Our preliminary research study helped our team to understand what women all around us were eager to have us know. Their experiences of suffering and of physical and psychological danger were being ignored. Their efforts to communicate critical information about their bodies, their emotional strengths, and their vulnerabilities were not being heard, leaving them and their babies in danger.

The transcriptions of the interviews with the women in our preliminary study who experienced a traumatic birth yielded hundreds of pages of narratives. I was eager to analyze the data, the women's words, and to learn from them what factors contributed to making their childbirth experience traumatic. What I was not prepared for was the impact of the women's words on me.

As our research team read and re-read each transcript, subjecting each one to an ethnographic analysis, which attempted to bring into focus the most important aspects of the childbirth experience, I found myself drawn into the life of the traumatic experience so deeply that the psychological pain threatened to overwhelm me. The beginning lines of a poem by Emily Dickinson expresses the feeling aroused in me in the presence of the women's stories:

"There is a pain—so utter—It swallows substance up—"

No matter how my colleagues sought to reassure me that we could manage the data with objectivity, I came to understand that there was something so deeply disturbing to me in hearing these women's stories that I could not pretend to objectivity. Since I had been working with

CHAPTER 2: SOMETHING IS TERRIBLY WRONG

accounts of traumatic suffering of every kind and description for over twenty years, this took me by surprise. I had never before felt so personally impacted. What was it about these stories, these women and their words, that was so distressing to me?

For many years I could not answer that question. I understood with my intuition, however, that to proceed further, to immerse myself more deeply into the women's experiences of trauma, presented a certain kind of danger for me that I was not ready to confront or master. Just as I was not ready at the time of the search to understand why the encounter with William moved me so deeply, I was not ready to face the experiences of invalidation, pain, and fear described so poignantly by the women in our study. So I set aside the research project, leaving others to complete the analysis of the data. I consulted from afar. Although the copies of the women's words remained carefully contained in my file drawers, their voices remained fresh in my heart through all these years.

As mentioned earlier, one cannot confront experiences of trauma until one is ready: until the right combination of companions, tools, and inner strength are present to withstand the difficulties of seeing the entire picture and finding its meaning and place within one's life. Such readiness is a matter of subjective evaluation that cannot and should not be overridden or hastened by the efforts of others. It may take months, or years, or a lifetime to achieve such readiness, if at all.

My response to this research into the nature of traumatic birth experience is similar to my response to the search for William. When I saw William face-to-face, sitting utterly alone in the dark woods, I recognized in his experience of aloneness a reflection of a very early experience of aloneness in my own life. Similarly, in the stories told by the women in our study who felt that their cries of alarm were not heard or given credence, I found a reflection of my own early-life experience of invalidation—invalidation of my awareness that something was terribly wrong. But what that "something" was I could not name. It was based on a feeling of anxiety that floated freely in our family and seemed somehow to circle around my mother. In the logic of the legacy of traumatic experience, my mother's sense of danger and dread became my sense of danger and foreboding: the two were inseparable. I would have to understand both her experiences and my own to learn what had gone so wrong.

An Accident

Regardless of whether a person's perception of things going terribly wrong occurs at the outset of traumatic injury—as a harbinger of mounting danger—or long after the "event" of the trauma has passed, the invalidation of a person's perception that danger is at hand can have profoundly distressing and disturbing consequences. Oliver Sacks' story of his traumatic injury and equally traumatic treatment in a London hospital provides a dramatic illustration of the critical importance of validation in both the prevention of and healing from trauma.

On a mild and cloudy summer morning in 1974, Oliver Sacks took off alone to hike a mountain that rose some 6,000 feet above a fjord and a small village in a rural area of Norway where he was vacationing. What began as a pleasurable holiday hike became, in a few short hours, an all-out struggle for survival. Sacks badly injured his leg in a fall before he had attained the summit. Desperate to reach the safety of the few houses at the foot of the mountain before nightfall, Sacks slid on his hands and back down the steep, rocky slopes for over seven hours. His torn and useless leg registered the pain of every inch of the descent.

But for all of his agonizing effort, Sacks was unable to come within sight or shouting distance of help. As night closed in, covering the mountain in darkness, he lay helpless and exhausted, far above the village. As cold and darkness began to take away all hope of surviving the night, he was found, miraculously, entirely by accident, by reindeer hunters who had come to set up their camp on the mountain.

CHAPTER 2: SOMETHING IS TERRIBLY WRONG

What occurred in the following weeks in a London hospital where he was taken for care was a nightmare of experience that was every bit as terrifying, if not more so, than what Sacks had endured after his fall on the mountain. He was, in fact, traumatized again in the course of his medical treatment—treatment which did not take into account his own perception of the devastating nature of his wounds.

When Sacks fell, he tore the quadriceps muscles of his upper leg from their attachment to the knee, rendering his leg entirely useless. The nerves in the affected area were torn and damaged also, creating a cacophony of pain. Surgery was required to re-attach the parts of his leg. The view of the surgeon and the medical staff was confident and straightforward. When the surgeon spoke to Sacks of what they would do, he said: "The parts of your leg have become detached; we re-attach them; that's all there is to it."

But that was not all there was to it. Although from the surgeon's vantage point the operation was a success, for Sacks it was a disaster that resulted in unspeakable terror. Although he had no medical explanation with which to validate his self-perception, soon after the surgery he knew with utmost clarity that "there was something amiss, something deeply the matter, something with no precedent in my entire experience." His dreams and his waking perception told him that he had "lost" his leg. He no longer had an internal image of it. His leg was no longer a part of his body. He could not move it. In fact, his leg fell off the bed without his awareness or control, causing his nurses to chastise him.

For Sacks, his leg simply did not exist in his internal frame of reference—not in his mind, not in his nerve pathways, not in his feelings, not in his spirit. In the process of the injury and surgery, his leg had "died." He was left with profound confusion and grief. That he was himself a physician—even a neurologist—did not help him to understand his experience or to cope with it. As he explains, he was a patient and could not be a doctor to himself.

Unfortunately, Mr. Swan, his surgeon, was not able to be the doctor that Sacks needed either. When Sacks told him of his inability to perceive or recognize his injured leg, the doctor replied: "Nonsense, Sacks...there's nothing the matter. Nothing at all. Nothing to be worried about. Nothing at all!...You're completely mistaken...there's nothing wrong with the leg." And again, when Sacks tried, some time later, to explain to the resident physician that "the leg doesn't feel right," the doctor replied: "This is very vague and subjective. Not the sort of thing we can be concerned with....Sacks, you're unique....I've never heard anything like this from a patient before."

The medical and nursing staff essentially looked upon Sacks as a recalcitrant patient. It made no sense to them that Sacks had "lost" his leg, when surgically it had been so successfully put back together, and it was quite clearly, to them, a part of him.

Because "there was no construct," Sacks explains, in science, psychology or philosophy, with which to explain or understand the subjective experience of his injury and post-operative recovery, Sacks came to view himself as unique. He had lost his sense of meaningful connection with himself and others. The fact that both doctors and nurses failed to heed his warning that something was terribly wrong served to invalidate his experience of himself as a reliable, credible observer and interpreter of his own experience. This, in turn, led him to descend into an abyss of darkness, silence, and utter aloneness: an experience, as he defined it, of trauma.

The famous Russian neurologist A. R. Luria was a mentor and revered elder whom Sacks later consulted about his trauma. In a letter he wrote to Sacks, Luria highlighted the defining aspect of Sacks' traumatic experience. The "alienation" of his injured leg from the rest of his body, and his feeling of disconnection of his body from his sense of a cohesive self— "cannot be measured or filmed or seen, it can only be reported, by the experiencer, a conscious human observer." Luria affirms that because of the essential subjectivity of the traumatic experience the wounded per-

CHAPTER 2: SOMETHING IS TERRIBLY WRONG

son finds him- or herself entirely alone. He is at the mercy of others who may or may not understand and validate the frightening dislocation of self that has occurred.

This is the heart of the problem for those who attempt to express their subjective experience. As with Sacks, or the women in childbirth, and countless others who stand at the precipice of traumatic experience, when objective observers (such as medical staff, friends, or psychiatrists) cannot see, film, or measure the difficulty reported by the injured, suffering person, they tend to discount and discredit it as meaningless, allowing the "subject" to descend alone into the gaping hole of traumatic experience.

It was many weeks after his surgery before Sacks found the validation he needed. It came first in the empathic understanding of patients in the rehabilitation center where he was transferred from the hospital. With them he was no longer "strange" and "unique"; he was one of many injured people who were trying to become whole again. Some of the patients there had experiences that were similar enough to give Sacks some hope that he was not crazy after all.

Finally, some two months after his surgery, Sacks sought and found an orthopedist who "listened, with perfect concentration and courtesy" to the complete story of the trauma he had endured: physical, emotional, mental, and spiritual. Finally, this doctor explained that the internal experience of alienation, the loss of the part of the body that Sacks had experienced "is a common phenomenon." He said: "I often see it in my patients, and I warn them beforehand." For the first time since his injury, Sacks felt respected and understood.

A person who struggles with grave injury is both fragile and fragmented. He needs to see in the eyes of the physician or healer a vision of wholeness, of integrity, and of meaning. To be invalidated is to be made an invalid; it is to be encouraged into helplessness and despair.

Sacks' encounter with this "masterful" physician caused him to wonder if much of his terrible experience of fragmentation and loss of cohesion could have been averted if this man had been his surgeon. Not only would he have been warned in advance about the frightening feeling of alienation from his body and from himself that could occur, but his perception that something was very wrong would have been validated and measures would have been taken to discuss with him the real problems caused by the injury, to reassure him and to decrease his isolation.

As Sacks explains, this was an immensely complex neuropsychological phenomenon that he experienced in the course of his injury and recovery. Although it was not uncommon, it had not been studied nor was it discussed in the literature of neurology or psychology. Thus, the orthopedist's suggestion to Sacks that he might want to describe his experience in a book had serious intent. It also served to validate a core part of Sacks' identity that had been crushed: that of being a credible narrator of his own experience, as well as being a scientist who could study and report on what he had gone through to benefit others.

Once again, however, there is a question of readiness. Sacks was deeply wounded by this simple accident. While his leg healed, after much rehabilitation and hard work, his psychological structure required a different and lengthy healing process. Such an experience of invalidation of one's self-awareness and truthfulness is not easily healed. Like the women who experienced trauma in childbirth, Sacks thought of himself (in the context of this accident and injury) as "hysterical" and "mad." It took a very long time, some of which was spent in simply "forgetting" the entire experience, to regain the confidence and integrity that he had lost as a result of his accident and its aftermath. It would be ten years before he published *A Leg to Stand On*, his deeply personal and dramatic account of his injuries and recovery, combined with his medical research and theoretical formulations regarding the neuropsychological phenomenon he had endured.

CHAPTER 3

How Connections Are Lost

"One looks into the abyss in order to see beyond it."
—ROBERT JAY LIFTON

So much of what we ordinarily think of and talk about as "trauma" is really what happens leading into and going out of the traumatic experience: the beginning and ending parts of the overall process of trauma. The trauma itself, that place in the center—in the eye of the storm—almost defies description. It is a place where everything and nothing co-exist; where there is too much and nothing at all.

To describe an experience of such profound loss of all that serves to keep us in touch not only with the world around us, our place in time and space, but also with the reality of our own being, presents a challenge for all who have experienced trauma and to those who seek to bear witness to their wounds. No matter how difficult the task, however, it is important to understand the core of traumatic experience in order to understand and care for oneself as a survivor and to offer understanding and care to others who have managed to endure.

The Traumatic Process

Traumatic experience may begin with a physical injury or an emotional wound or both at once. The natural progression of the traumatic process may take place in a matter of moments (as in a car crash, medical crisis, explosion, or violent event) or over the course of days or even years (as in domestic violence, war, or imprisonment). Regardless of the event initiating the traumatic process, its progress—if uninterrupted—compromises all aspects of a person's life. Connections with life-supporting structures both within and external to the sufferer erode, then finally break.

To form a picture of the progressive deconstruction engendered by the traumatic process, imagine first a universe of color and light. The self, yourself perhaps, is at the very center, colored a vibrant, glowing green. Surrounding the self are orbs of people and spheres of influence and interdependence, colored in blues and reds and myriad other hues. These spheres and planet-others circulating around the self include the natural world and all aspects of the environment: culture (including art, traditions, literature, music, and ritual), the infrastructure of social life (car, TV and Internet, a social group, insurance providers). Closer in, surrounding the self, there are the more intimate connections with work colleagues, extended family, physician, and supportive groups. And finally, closest of all, are loved ones: an intimate partner, parents, a pet, and others. Holding together this rich system of interconnections is a kind of connective tissue, colored a brilliant primary yellow, which is made up of activity, energy, engagement, and reciprocal exchange.

As the traumatic process proceeds, the connection between the self and each of these external resources becomes loosened and is torn. Finally the connections fail altogether, leaving only the blackness of space where once there were vibrant others in a sea of activity. When those vital external connections are lost, the individual is left floating alone in a dark place, with no references to anchor the self.

At the same time that the connections with the external world are diminishing or being torn apart, the inner structures of the self begin to lose their connection to one another. The vibrant activity and energy that has held the parts of the self together are compromised and diminished

CHAPTER 3: HOW CONNECTIONS ARE LOST

also and are finally extinguished as the traumatic process moves forward. This loss of internal connections renders inoperable the capacities of the brain, the complexities and modulation of emotional response, the certainties of spiritual understanding, and the body's ability to function. The result is that the mind can no longer interpret messages from the body, nor can the body receive information from the brain. Feelings become detached from the events and experiences that gave rise to them. Fear, which once belonged to an event, now floods everything. Reason cannot mediate the impact of feelings. The connective tissue that held all these functions together is shredded and lost, leaving behind nothing but black holes. The self is entirely bereft of references, within or outside of itself, so that time and space no longer have meaning nor provide an anchor.

This is a picture described by many who have descended into the abyss of trauma and lived to recount their experiences.

A different, less visual way of describing this is provided by Mordechai Benyakar, a psychiatrist, who, together with a team of Israeli researchers, has defined the traumatic process as a structural collapse: a systemic deconstruction that occurs as the traumatic process overwhelms the ability to function. They explain:

— *Trauma is an experience of structural collapse along all planes of reference which may be life-threatening to the individual, family or group. If trauma is to be used, not just as a vague historical rudiment, but as a viable, meaningful...concept, it must convey its original metaphorical essence; the notion of injury and discontinuity, which, in its psychological context should capture the sense of irreparable tear of self and reality.*

What causes the traumatic experience is not merely the presence of mounting unacceptable emotions, but the perception of the diminishing ability, or even loss of ability to perform the essential autonomous functions that define the human system. The central feature of the traumatic experience is the final horrible "realization" that the rules that define the individual's identity and reality are not operational any more. In structural terms, this means that wholeness, transformation, and self-regulation are no longer feasible, and hence, the very existence of the structure itself is questionable, incomprehensible, or non-existent.

Hypothermia, a condition resulting from the loss of core body heat, offers an excellent example of the process of deconstruction of core functions of the self common to most experiences of profound trauma. Hypothermia results from a convergence of circumstances leading to a critical loss of one's ability to maintain life-sustaining functions. Eventually, if not interrupted, it will lead to death. The wound or trauma in this instance is not inflicted by another person or by oneself. It is delivered by the indifference of nature—by cold.

Hypothermia is a medical problem that can affect a wide range of people, from the frail elderly who live in poorly heated dwellings to Boy Scouts out for a Sunday hike. It is not an uncommon affliction among climbers scaling high mountain peaks. Mountaineers often describe the hypothermic process as a "siren call of the snows" in which the exhausted climber is lured toward the peaceful sleep of death. Many people experience a similar resignation to death as traumatic loss overwhelms their ability to resist their own extinction.

In the process of hypothermia, as the body's core temperature drops, the external world fades from awareness. The demands of the heart, the lungs, and other vital organs take precedence over all other demands. Fingers don't count, toes aren't needed, arms aren't essential, legs become an awkward nuisance. The brain quickly loses its ability to process information, and judgment suffers. The voices of friends become distant and seem unreal. At the same time, one's own inner voice plays tricks—giving false assurances and lies—trying to outwit the danger that is overtaking the mind and body. The sense of time and place lose their meaning.

CHAPTER 3: HOW CONNECTIONS ARE LOST

And so the diminution proceeds, inexorably, until finally the connections with the reality of one's body, with one's mind and emotions, with one's companions, and with one's place in the world are broken. For life to continue, the process must be interrupted by internal or external intervention, or one dies.

The story of Joe Simpson's survival after a climbing fall in remote Andean mountains provides a dramatic example of the course of the traumatic process.

Touching the Void

For Joe Simpson, the siren voice of hypothermia—with its sure promise of death—was always present as he struggled with a shattered leg down the side of Siula Grande, through blizzards, to reach the safety of his camp miles below. Simpson, a British mountaineer, has provided a harrowing account of his descent of the mountain and of his descent into traumatic experience in his book and recent film, *Touching the Void*. His story is important to an exploration of traumatic experience because of his ability to recount not only the physiological dangers and hardships he endured but also his ability to speak honestly of the metaphysical crisis that resulted from his confrontation with his utter aloneness.

In June of 1985, soon after summiting the 21,000-foot mountain Siula Grande, located in the remote Peruvian Andes, Simpson and his climbing partner Simon Yates crossed a razor-thin ridge with fragile cornices and sheer drops of thousands of feet on either side. Desperate to get off the ridge, Joe began to descend a near-vertical ice wall. But his ice axe and hammer couldn't hold, and he fell onto the steep slope below, jamming his straight legs into the ice, then catapulting further down the slope. Miraculously, the suddenness and force of the fall didn't pull Simon off the ridge also. He was able to arrest Joe's fall with the rope that bound their fate together.

As Joe righted himself and surveyed his injury, it was as though his self-appraisal presented a death sentence. The impact of the fall had forced the bones of his lower leg up through his knee, rupturing the knee joint, tearing it to pieces, which rendered his leg entirely useless. It was unimaginable that he could descend the mountain with such an injury.

Simon climbed down to where Joe pressed his wounded body against the steep slope, and together they assessed their precarious position on the mountain and the extent of Joe's injury. Neither man held much hope that they could make it back to their camp many miles below. Simon set to work, however, to improvise a rope system with which to try to lower Joe and himself to safety.

With hands already frozen and temperatures near minus eighty degrees F in howling winds, Simon soon began the long process of lowering Joe, 300 feet at a time, the length of two ropes tied together, down the sheer ice walls and snow slopes toward the glacier below. With each release of the rope, Joe's broken leg crashed into the mountainside, setting off waves of unbearable agony.

Finally, after hours of excruciating effort for both men, with only a few hundred feet of descent remaining to reach the easier slope of the glacier below, Joe dropped out of sight over a ledge. Simon could not see Joe, nor could he hear him as Joe called to Simon in the storm. Joe was entirely helpless, dangling free in space at the end of the rope. Simon could not go to him; if he did, they both would fly off the face of the mountain.

In the continuing storm, with the dark and utter cold of night beginning to settle in, Simon finally realized that he could no longer hold onto the rope with his frozen hands. In addition, he was slowly sliding out of his belay seat dug into the snow and soon would topple off the slope himself. He knew it was beyond his ability to help Joe, who dangled in midair at the other end of the fragile line that connected them. He wasn't sure, in fact, that Joe was still alive, since Joe had stopped moving on the end of

CHAPTER 3: HOW CONNECTIONS ARE LOST

the rope a long time ago. And so Simon made a decision: he cut the rope that bound Joe and him together on the mountain. It was the only thing he knew to do.

Startled out of the lethargy of hypothermia and resignation to death, Joe cascaded in a free fall straight down the cliff face for more than one hundred feet—down into the open mouth of a waiting crevasse.

When he became conscious, Joe found himself splayed on an icy ledge some fifty feet deep in the crevasse; its walls of ice towered above him on all sides. He knew he could not climb them to free himself. He was too wounded. Alone, injured, frozen, and terrified—with no food, water, or heat source—Joe struggled against dread, despair, and death, all of which threatened to overwhelm him.

At this moment in time, Joe explains, he felt that his faith, or lack thereof, was being challenged. Since he had not believed in God prior to this time, he wondered if the extremity of the situation would bring forth in him a sudden awakening to belief. He wryly comments that it did not. He found no prayer coming from his lips, only expletives and self-criticism. There was no God, no climbing partner, no source of connection outside of himself to which he could turn for help. He was entirely alone.

Joe still had internal resources, however, that were not extinguished. At this time of greatest personal despair, as he meticulously explored the ice tomb in which he was trapped, he explored also the depths of himself: his terror, his rage, and his determination to live. His stubbornness, a personal characteristic that at other times might have been an obstacle, was at this time a needed asset. Remarkably, he was able to tolerate intense self-examination and to arrive at a critical decision—to go even deeper—to descend further into the crevasse in order to try to live.

The decision to venture further into the black place that yawned below him—into the icy, unfathomed depths—served as an unwitting metaphor for Joe's journey not only to survive physically but to endure emotionally as well. "You have to make a decision," Joe explains, with utmost simplicity. To do nothing at all is to surrender to the inevitability of danger and certainly to die.

To descend into the unknown depths of the crevasse was counterintuitive. The alternative, however—to wait for his life to end, entrapped by ice—was unthinkable. His inner voice of determination and desire to live was still strong. His body's skills to think and move were still available. The seductive call of hypothermia was not strong enough yet to lure him to give up.

After lowering himself more than eighty feet deeper into the total darkness of the icy cavern, Joe reached another precarious shelf of snow and ice on which to rest. He was almost at the end of his rope—literally, not as a figure of speech. As he cautiously surveyed his surroundings, he saw a faint glimmer of light some distance above him, coming through a small hole in a side-sloping wall, at an angle to the main shaft. With enormous effort he climbed and clawed his way up the slope toward the light, then punched his way through the hole to collapse onto the side of the mountain, in sunshine.

Exhausted and severely dehydrated, Joe began a new phase of his saga of survival. For hours that became days he crawled on his stomach and slid on his back, inching his way down the icy glacier, navigating a labyrinthine course through dozens of crevasses that opened on every side of his path. Becoming delirious, sometimes hallucinating images and sounds, he lurched across the boulder-filled moraine that stretched for miles in the direction toward the camp from which he had set out on this terrible journey many days before.

Finally, after seven days in the mountains, four of which he suffered with the constant agony of his wrecked leg, with exposure to extremes of temperatures and storms, with little water and no food—his body consuming itself instead—Joe began to lose the internal mental structures that had kept him oriented to time and place. He knew deeply that he no longer had the capacity to save himself, to intervene on his own behalf. It

CHAPTER 3: HOW CONNECTIONS ARE LOST

would, in fact, be a relief to die, though he could not yet release his hold on life.

In extremis, Joe cried out Simon's name, one last time, asserting his need for connection, not to be left utterly alone, and his absolute need for someone to come to help him at a time when he could no longer help himself. Perhaps his cry to Simon was also a final effort to assert that he still existed as a sentient being: the sound of his voice attesting "I am!"

As he lay among boulders, delirious, shriveled, hardly conscious, he recalls thinking that even if he found the camp, Simon would probably have left by this time. Joe writes:

— *The cold was taking me again. I felt its insidious touch on my back. I wouldn't survive this night, that was for sure, but I no longer cared. The notions of living or dying had long since become tangled. The past days merged into a blur of real events and madness, and now I seemed fixed in a limbo between the two. Alive, dead, was there that much difference? I raised my head and howled a name into the darkness:*

"SIIIIIIIMMMMMMmmooooonnnn..."

The pleading in my head had become hysterical, and I heard a voice moaning in a cracked whisper, as if I were listening to someone else!

"Please be there...you must be there...help me."

The night remained black. Warm tears mingled with the cold melted snow on my face. I wanted it to end. I felt destroyed. For the first time in many days I accepted that I had finally come to the end of my strength. I needed someone, anyone. This dark night-storm was taking me and I had no more will to resist. I cried for many things, but mostly for not having someone to be with in this awful night. I let my head fall to my chest, ignored the darkness, and let the anger and pain weep. It was too much for me. I just couldn't keep on; too much of everything.

As he narrates this final experience of his struggle to hold on to life, to reach help, Joe explains—in his film narration of the story—that it was at this point, when there was no answer to his calls for help, only silence and the continued howling of the wind, that a certain threshold was crossed. On screen, with his face and eyes filling the frame, he states quietly, thoughtfully, as though for the first time giving full recognition to the truth of his own words: "I lost something then. I lost—me."

Hearing himself speak these words, tears appear unbidden: his body's testament to the terrible, irreparable loss he had suffered.

Miraculously, Simon was there, and he heard Joe's voice above the screaming storm. He raced from the safety of his tent at the camp and searched for Joe in the dark among the boulders many yards away. When he found Joe, Simon was stunned to see his friend almost lifeless—yet alive. He had been certain that Joe was dead, that he could not have survived all those days and nights of cold and snow and injury. He cradled him in his arms and reassured him that he was there, that he would keep him safe, and that he would help him. And he did.

In many accounts of trauma in which survivors speak of descending into the core of suffering, they speak of their aloneness as the central, unbearable aspect of the experience. It is not the prospect of death, nor pain, nor fear which consumes those horrific moments: it is the sense of utter aloneness. In the Christian tradition, accounts of Jesus' life, recorded in the books of Matthew and Mark of the Bible, tell that at his crucifixion, "in the ninth hour," just as death was overtaking his wounded, exhausted body, Jesus cried out: "My God, my God, why hast thou forsaken me?" His dreadful cry of abandonment, of utter aloneness, was mirrored in the heavens. The sun cast no light, and there was utter darkness as he spoke these same words a second time; then he died. The place of silence and darkness into which Jesus descended at the end of his life was made complete when he was sealed in a tomb. Yet, from this silent center, new life began.

The Hole in Experience

When all connections are lost, when the hope that someone will hear the cry for help is extinguished, and when the body's resources are depleted beyond self-repair, there is both an end and a beginning present at once. In so many autobiographical narratives of trauma, people who have suffered widely diverse events record a similar view, using similar words to describe the core of their traumatic experience. They speak of a great hole, a hiatus, a gap, in which there is no feeling, no thought, no sensation. In the center there is absence and presence all at once. There is no story in the center, only in the leading in and the going out of the void. A few examples may help to illustrate this complex phenomenon.

When Gretel Ehrlich was struck by lightning, on an August afternoon in 1991 as she walked in a high mountain meadow near her ranch in Montana, she describes that she fell into an ocean of unconsciousness: she fell into a hiatus or gap in experience, in which her life and her death coexisted in the same moment. For many months after her injury, Ehrlich returned to this territory of death-in-life, as her body struggled to regain its equilibrium and her heart searched for a way to maintain its rhythms and strength.

Reflecting on this aspect of her experience, Ehrlich refers to this transitional place as "that wandering state between life and death, confusion and enlightenment.... The past has just occurred, and the future has not yet happened."

The mountaineer Ruth Anne Kocour confronted that transitional space at the heart of trauma in a dream. Trapped for two weeks by blizzards on the upper slopes of Denali, unsure of her ability to survive, yet determined not to give in to her fear and dread, Kocour saw in her dream what she could not allow herself to imagine in her waking hours. In her journal she wrote:

— *Last night a woman came to visit me in my dreams. She stood just out of my reach holding warm blankets and beckoning to me. I have no doubt in my mind that I was looking at death—in this case a seductress, teasing, enticing....I am beginning to believe that existence on earth isn't limited to a solid state. There's a transitional place, a real place—a gray area, if you will—where life and death are closer than I'd previously imagined. Here, on this mountain, I felt as if I were constantly straddling the line between the two. Maybe too much has been made of the distinction between life and death. Maybe it's only a subtle transition. Maybe there's nothing really to fear...maybe.*

Oliver Sacks also talks about this gap in experience at the heart of traumatic experience. He describes it as a limbo, a nothingness, a hell—a hole into which he plunged in the wake of the injury to his leg. He writes:

— *There was a gap—an absolute gap—between then and now; and in that gap, into the void, the former "I" had vanished—the "I" who could thoughtlessly stand, run and walk....Into that gap, that void, outside space and time, the reality and possibilities of the leg had passed, and disappeared.*

    All the cognitive and intellectual and imaginative powers which had previously aided me in exploring different neurological lands were wholly useless, meaningless, in the limbo of Nowhere. I had fallen off the map, the world, of the knowable. I had fallen out of space, and out of time too. Nothing could happen, ever, any more. Intelligence, reason, sense, meant nothing. Memory, imagination, hope, meant nothing. I had lost everything which afforded a foothold before. I had entered, willy-nilly, a dark night of the soul.

I felt that my own story had the shape of such a universal existential experience, the journey of a soul into the underworld and back, a spiritual drama—on a neurological basis.

The progressive loss of connection with one's place in the world, with caring others, with a sense of time and space, and with the continuity of one's sense of identity and cohesiveness defines traumatic experience.

Another Kind of Death

Emerging from the concentration camps of Europe after the Second World War, many survivors described the extremes of suffering they experienced and witnessed in the camps. Primo Levi spoke of two kinds of death he saw: "The first," he said, "occurred when a person surrendered to despair; he would die. And if he didn't surrender to despair, but survived as an angry, vicious animal, stealing crusts of bread and bowls of soup from others, then he died inside as a human being."

Henry Krystal's therapeutic work with many holocaust survivors, as well as his psychiatric study of human personality, affirmed Levi's observation, and Krystal concluded that "the beginning of the traumatic process is the surrender to inevitable danger, which if not interrupted may lead to psychogenic death." Such "danger" may be understood not only as an external threat but also as an internal perception of the loss of one's identity, of all that one understands as defining one's self and one's competence and confidence to survive.

Not only the horrors of war, but also accidents and cruelties of life can cause a person to give up on the struggle to live. Krystal gives an example of a small child who has been abandoned by the roadside. At first the child will anticipate the return of the parent. Slowly, however, hope fades. Even the memory of the person who cared for him fades. Eventually the child will "surrender" to his awareness that no one is coming to care for him. He will not be able to help himself to live. He will fail to thrive and die. This was the tragedy of so many, young and old, in the concentration camps and ghettoes of WWII. It is a continuing tragedy lived out in our nursing homes and prisons, in present-day American-run concentration camps where men and boys who are called "hostile combatants" are held, and in ordinary homes where domestic abuse is an inevitable danger.

Another kind of death, a dying inside, or loss of ability to connect with human feelings, is sometimes seen in a person's deep withdrawal into a perpetual state of numbness, a death-in-life. Two movies in particular, *The Pawnbroker* and *The Fisher King*, offer accurate and dramatic depictions of the extremes of numbing and withdrawal caused by traumatic suffering. In these films, the central characters, Sol Nazerman and a man simply named Parry, appear to be very different from each other in the ways their personalities are shaped by their traumatic experiences, yet they are responding to very similar life events. Each man was forced to witness the brutal murder of his beloved wife. Each man was then locked away. Nazerman was interned in a death camp, Parry in a mental hospital. Both emerged as men without a past. Their memories were so unbearable that they could no longer be permitted into consciousness as a part of everyday life.

A person so profoundly wounded is vulnerable to flashbacks—sudden images, smells, sounds, or scenes from the forbidden past—which can send him rushing headlong into re-experiencing the entire traumatic event and feelings again in the present. It is horrifying and debilitating to be tossed from one life into another, without consent or control, only to have to reconstruct once again, in the aftermath, a life that is endurable.

In *The Fisher King* it becomes clear that Parry's story is only one of many, that wounded lives are a familiar part of our daily surroundings. But because such wounded people seem to be separate from us, responding to a different reality, or not responding at all, we turn away from them. To look, to listen, and to acknowledge their woundedness is to see the vulnerability of our own lives. And often they cannot tell us their own stories, even if we do want to hear, because each story is contained in that spaceless, timeless place of the void—the bardo, the gap at the heart of traumatic experience—where no words exist.

Suicide

Death itself, the final withdrawal or removal from life, may become the siren call to those who have suffered beyond their capacity to endure. Such a surrender might be called suicide; yet this term does not begin to describe the dilemma of the individual who finds himself trapped in a life of horror, horror in present suffering or the horror of remembering and reliving experience in which traumatic memories are played over and over like the endless looping of sound. This is the perfect tragic irony: that for some trauma survivors, the only hope left is the hope of death. Death, they believe, will bring an end to the trauma; then new life can begin.

In the narratives of some of the women who experienced childbirth as traumatic, this paradox was manifested in the statement: "I thought I was going to die....I wanted to die." It expressed the wish to be done with the agony, to be done with the traumatic experience as it was unfolding and engulfing them with suffering. This desperate solution—the thought of fending off the danger of trauma by dying—was described also by both Joe Simpson and Oliver Sacks in their accounts of their traumatic experiences.

In the context of traumatic suffering, this yearning for death is not the same as a wish to be done with life. In this instance, the suicidal wish gives expression to a desire, a hope to continue life, free from traumatic suffering, and free from reliving the traumatic experience.

Traumatic Grief

Grief is the expression of the loss of connection with a meaningful part of one's life, both internal and external. One can grieve the loss of connection with a part of one's body; and one can grieve the loss of the ability to think or to feel. As we hear from many individuals who find themselves confined to nursing homes, one can grieve the loss of autonomous function; and one can grieve the loss of one's sense of self, one's identity. Some people have documented the progress of Alzheimer's disease as it fragments their connections with self and the outside world, and they speak of the terrible grief they feel for the parts of themselves that are taken from them by the disease. One can also grieve the loss of a beloved, of one's home, of a pet, of employment, of community—all those structures and relationships which give texture and meaning to life. The measure and impact of a particular loss is subjective. Each person responds uniquely to his or her own loss.

Traumatic grief is found at the far end of a continuum of grief experiences. It is often precipitated by a loss that threatens the identity, integrity, sense of safety, and wholeness of the survivor. This can be most clearly seen in the death of a beloved. The more closely the life of the individual who dies is bound together with those who survive, the deeper may be the traumatic loss.

In the following story that was told to me by a colleague, we are introduced to an older woman who was struck down by the loss of her beloved husband. He did not die unexpectedly; however, their long marriage and love for each other made the woman's final loss of connection to their shared, intertwined lives an insupportable loss.

This story also offers a unique view of the force of compassionate response that is required to reach into the dark void of traumatic grief and bring the wounded person out to safety. Only after a person has been

CHAPTER 3: HOW CONNECTIONS ARE LOST

brought out of that place of nothingness, where all connections to self and others have been lost, can the long process of normal grieving begin to take place. This is the story of May and Edna, as May described it to me.

As bereavement counselor for her Hospice program, May was used to receiving calls from her team of nurses and aides. The number on her pager this day was from a team member who was at the home of an elderly gentleman being cared for in his last days of life by Hospice and family members. Since she was in the neighborhood, May decided to stop by to see what she could do to help.

What May found when she arrived at the small private home of the family was a scene of complete anguish and confusion. Family members were pounding on the door of the home, calling the name of the elderly man's wife. She was shut inside and would let no one in. Her husband of sixty years had died only a few hours before; he had been taken to the mortuary; his wife's grief seemed inconsolable.

May learned all of this from her co-worker who was trying to calm the family. All were concerned about the elderly wife who was alternately wailing with grief and mute with shock. From the sidewalk they could hear her cry: "Take me, take me with you!" May knew the woman, knew her to be a strong and devoted person who, no matter how she had tried to prepare for her husband's death, would be terribly wounded, like a giant redwood struck by lightning.

May made her way to the door and knocked. There was no sound. The silence now was almost more frightening than the loud sobbing that had come through the door a few moments before. She spoke to the door, quietly calling the woman's name: "Edna, Edna—It's me, May. I would like to come in." After long moments in which there was no answer from Edna, a family member lifted a small grandchild through an open kitchen window. Soon the front door opened, and as the boy ran out, May ventured into the home.

Inside the front room, darkened by drawn curtains, Edna sat slumped in a large chair, her husband's favorite chair. She was inert, mute, and her eyes stared blankly into distant space. For a moment May wondered if Edna had died also, in order to be with her husband, as if her love had been so strong as to will her body into joining him. Looking closely, however, May could see shallow breathing reflected in the slight movement of her hollow chest. Quietly she began to talk to Edna. She reassured her and soothingly sought to coax her into some connection. But Edna was firmly locked away. It was possible she might choose to stay there, forever.

Slowly, quietly, gently, May climbed into the chair with Edna. She took the old woman's body into her arms, their heads and breath touching softly. She rocked and crooned and talked of pain and loss and love. She talked of Harry, Edna's husband. She talked of their children and grandchildren. She talked and rocked and soothed and cradled the old woman's pain. And soon there were tears flowing down the two women's cheeks. They were joined in grief and remembering and in a deep connection with each other.

In a little while Edna's body grew soft and molded into May's arms. She began to breathe in long and regular sighs of loss. Her cold skin became warmer. May slipped to the floor and knelt in front of Edna, holding her hands and holding her with her kind eyes. She talked to Edna of what had transpired in the past few hours, helping to bring her back into the world of family and safety—into the beginning of a new life without her beloved husband.

CHAPTER 4

Energies to Survive

"Survival is as much a matter of grace as fight."
—GRETEL EHRLICH

If there is no one to find you, no one beside you—to reach inside and pull you from the void—what forces can a person draw on to emerge from traumatic experience?

In any exploration of the internal resources and interventions a person may use to bring him- or herself through the dark center of trauma, it is necessary to consider not just the practical solutions that have helped people in extreme situations; it is also important to explore experiences that may be referred to as metaphysical and spiritual. These terms may seem vague and perhaps confusing when put next to terms such as "strategy," "plans," or "solutions." However, stories of traumatic injury, suffering, grief, and survival are replete with references to experiences that cannot be explained in scientific or practical terms but which represent a crucial aspect of some people's ability to survive.

Many survivors refer to a felt impulse of life: an energy of life that insists itself into the black hole of hopelessness and physical injury, and—like a match—strikes a spark with which new life may be kindled. They use words such as "grace," "miracle," "spirit," and "soul" to describe an experience that defies words.

For instance, in her book *A Match to the Heart*—in which she describes her recovery from having been struck by lightning—Gretel Ehrlich writes that "Survival is as much a matter of grace as fight." The very act of breathing in—inspiration—especially those first breaths that one takes after the body has been struck down by calamity—can be understood, she says, as "the taking in of divinity....As it moves through, it becomes a spark...."

In his study and teaching of comparative mythology, Joseph Campbell was able to unhook these powerful words, such as "grace" and "spirit," from specific traditions, religions or cultures, to provide a rich, cross-cultural context for understanding their central meaning to human experience. Of particular interest to me as I explore experiences and meanings of profound trauma is Campbell's discussion of the symbolic precursors and western Christian meanings attributed to the Grail, as object and as legend. Campbell explains that the Grail may be understood as the symbol of an energizing force. It represents the source from which life proceeds, for which one yearns and toward which one reaches for new creation in the wake of collapse.

As Campbell notes, the Grail has been referred to in legends as an "inexhaustible source, a cauldron, in depths of the unconscious, from which emerge the energies of life." This place in the center, this source of life, was referred to by T.S. Eliot as "the still point of the turning world, where motion and stasis are together, the hub where the movement of time and the stillness of eternity are together."

In the center of the storm, in the center of traumatic experience—in that moment of stillness, in the gap or the hole in which time and space no longer have reference and the end and the beginning are joined—there exists a source of life and energy. What enables one to reach out and join with that "inexhaustible source of energy" is as mysterious as the energy of life itself. How are new connections forged in the darkness and dread at the heart of traumatic loss?

CHAPTER 4: ENERGIES TO SURVIVE

Creating New Connections

It's no secret that many of us talk to ourselves all the time: chattering, bossing, consoling, reminding, and teasing. At times we can be heard to exclaim: "Good job!" or, "You fool!" even though it's only oneself who is receiving such praise or condemnation. So it's not surprising that such intense discussions with oneself might occur in times of extreme stress and hardship. Such a projection of oneself—throwing outward into the world one's own character—as if we actually belonged "out there"—may serve a very important life-sustaining function for the person who is mired in traumatic suffering.

Many who have survived terrible trauma have described a phenomenon in which their own voice takes on a presence of its own. Often called "the voice" by survivors, this observing "other presence" may take on the role of physician, clinically assessing injuries, diagnosing difficulties, and prescribing remedies. "The voice" may argue for pressing forward, taking one more step. It may argue for stopping. It cajoles and bargains and admonishes. It is a helper, a foil, and an essential companion. When it falls silent, fear and utter aloneness take its place.

Words from Afar

Another sort of companion or internal presence that may serve to forestall or lighten the impact of the solitude of traumatic experience is found in remembered characters and words of poems and stories. In many accounts of traumatic suffering, people recall that poetry, myths, and tales played an important role in their efforts to endure. Remembered words and images provide a link to a world outside of the traumatic experience. They remind the lonely, terrified person that others have traveled this territory of suffering before and have lived to write about it.

During the eight years of his imprisonment in the former Soviet Union, Natan Sharansky relied on this connection with others through remembered verses and stories. He felt an obligation, he explains, to act with integrity in his own world of suffering in order to honor those whose words he cherished as companions in suffering. In this "reverse connection," as he calls it, he experienced a powerful obligation to persevere and to endure.

Memories of favorite lines and verses from literature also help to remind the isolated person of a time that came before the suffering in which they encountered and memorized these words. To have this small connection with the continuity of oneself is a precious occurrence in the life of traumatic experience, which by definition takes away time and continuity.

Visions

Many people conjure images of the "other" as a source of encouragement, of care, even of need when no one is in fact present. Accounts of those who have survived harrowing experiences—whether on a mountain, in a prison, or lost in the desert—describe a strong feeling of like-mind with another. This imagined or remembered identification with another person serves as a source of strength and a clear representation of "normal" life: of familiar people and events that might occur in one's everyday life that are separate from the present disaster. Many survivors describe also states of altered consciousness, a dream-state, in which they experience the strong presence of a beloved other: a best friend, a husband, a mother, or even oneself.

Approaching the end of his strength and the end of his ability to endure, Joe Simpson experienced changes in his consciousness. He developed, for a short time, a vivid certainty that his climbing partner Simon and their camp-mate Richard were present with him as he struggled across the boulder-strewn moraine of Siula Grande to find his base camp. He was comforted by their presence and believed that they didn't reveal themselves to him in person because they didn't want him to be ashamed of the

CHAPTER 4: ENERGIES TO SURVIVE

terrible state he was in. His mind would try to find any reason to explain why they didn't come to help him, even though he was sure they were watching him from close by. Simpson explained: "I was just glad that they were there and someone knew I wasn't dead."

To maintain connection with another person who could bear witness to the fact that he was still alive was the primary need expressed in Simpson's imagined creation of the presence of his friends. It was his way of gaining some certainty that his worst fear had not yet come true: he would not die alone.

Another example of the kind of "vision" that a person creates in the extremes of traumatic experience to assist him- or herself in the struggle to survive is found in the story of Aron Ralston, the young outdoorsman and adventurer. In April 2003, during a solo recreational climbing trip into Blue John Canyon, a remote slot canyon in southern Utah, an 800-pound boulder crushed Ralston's right hand firmly against the canyon wall. For five days he struggled alone to find a way to release his arm from the weight of the boulder, to save himself. Finally, having exhausted his meager supply of food and water, as well as his alternatives to freeing himself, Ralston slipped into a trance. In this altered state, he left the confines of the canyon and found himself in a living room. A little boy greeted him. Defying the reality of his true situation, he used two arms, one missing a hand, to lift the boy up. He knew the child was his own and that he was viewing his future.

When the image collapsed and Ralston returned to the horror of his entrapment, he was nevertheless changed by the experience. He explains in his journal notes: "Despite having already come to accept that I will die where I stand before help arrives, now I believe I will live. That belief, that boy, changes everything for me."

The vision roused Ralston, at least for a time, from lethargy and defeat. It gave him a past and a future. All that remained was to endure and survive the present.

In the story of Beck Weathers, a physician and mountaineer, one is able to look deeply into that place in the center of trauma, to witness the energy of life making itself known and to marvel that a person so deeply wounded can survive. Once again, it was the vision of a beloved other, in fact three others—his wife, his daughter, and his son—that pulled Weathers from the depths of hypothermic coma and impelled him to struggle blindly toward safety.

Beck Weathers was left alone to die two separate times as storms raged around him on Mt. Everest in the spring of 1996. His story is now legend. He has written a book, *Left for Dead*, and given many public talks about his experiences. Many others, mountaineers and journalists, have added their own perspectives in books, articles, and films that chronicle the terrible events that occurred on Mt. Everest that spring. A fractured climbing community continues to try to puzzle together the facts and meanings from a mountaineering disaster that claimed nine lives in just a few days.

At the heart of Weathers' story is a miracle, the word he uses to describe his experience. Medicine and common sense said it was not possible for Weathers to live. His core body temperature would have registered extreme hypothermia, had such measurements been possible where he lay on the side of the mountain at 26,000 feet above sea level, in what is called "the death zone." His extremities were frozen into blocks of ice. His heart rate and breathing were barely detectable to the other climbers who passed by and left him for dead. But he would not die. He explains:

— *About four in the afternoon, Everest time—twenty-two hours into the storm—the miracle occurred.... The miracle was a quiet thing: I opened my eyes and was given a chance to try.*

CHAPTER 4: ENERGIES TO SURVIVE

Somewhere in the midst of all this came another shock—my epiphany. Suddenly, my family appeared in my mind's eye—Peach [his wife], Bub and Meg [his teenage children]....My subconscious summoned them into vivid focus, as if they might at any moment speak to me. I knew at that instant, with absolute clarity, that if I did not stand at once, I would spend an eternity on that spot.

Even though I was prepared to die, I just wasn't ready.

I am neither churchly nor a particularly spiritual person, but I can tell you that some force within me rejected death at the last moment and then guided me, blind and stumbling—quite literally a dead man walking—into camp and the shaky start of my return to life.

After raising himself from the snow and ice, Weathers began to make his way down the mountain. As both sunlight and his endurance waned and as he began to realize that he might not make it to High Camp and help, he describes being "overwhelmed by an enormous, encompassing sense of melancholy. That I would not say good-bye to my family...was just not acceptable."

Other aspects of Weathers' nightmare story on Everest—which includes a second time in which he was left for dead, even while other climbers moved around him in camp—will be discussed later (in Chapter 8) in the context of how help is offered or withheld from people who are in the deep center of traumatic experience, whether physical or psychological.

One final story is offered now to illustrate the creative imagining of the presence of an important "other" who augments a person's determination to survive circumstances of extreme physical, emotional, and spiritual degradation. From the cold, vertiginous landscape of the mountains, we move to the horizontal, barren landscape of the deserts of Libya, some seventy-five years ago.

Antoine de Saint-Exupéry began his career as a pilot in 1926 for a private airline that was the predecessor of the French Aeropostale, delivering the mail from Southern France to French West Africa and pioneering new routes across the Pyrenees and even to the Andes. In his famous story, "Prisoners of the Sand," recounted in his book *Wind, Sand and Stars*, Saint-Exupéry narrates his near-death experience in the desert, one of several he survived during the course of his aviation adventures.

Saint-Exupéry tells of how he and his co-pilot Prevot crashed in the Libyan desert, off-course from their flight plan, with no supplies and no idea in what direction lay human civilization. After having marched across the desert for forty miles, sometimes in circles, always lost, with no water, a striking vision presented itself to him. Saint-Exupéry writes:

> — *I was haunted by a vision of my wife's eyes under the halo of her hat. Of her face I could see only the eyes, questioning me, looking at me yearningly....Every time I saw those yearning eyes it was as if a flame were searing me. They were like a scream for help, like the flares of a sinking ship....I was perfectly ready to fall asleep, whether for a night or for eternity....the peace of sleep! But that cry that would be sent up at home, that great wail of desolation—that was what I could not bear....*

This is not an image of a comforting other but one of urgent need and grief. It served to give reason and meaning to Saint-Exupéry's struggle to survive. It reminded the numb aviator that he was firmly connected to another by feelings of love and responsibility. Even if he could no longer experience feelings of his own, he could be moved, impelled to movement, by the image of his wife's anguish. To strive to go toward his wife, toward the sounds and image of her grief was, he stated, a response to "a universal impulse."

CHAPTER 4: ENERGIES TO SURVIVE

The Power of Music

Most often we think of music as a form of stimulation that comes to us from some source outside ourselves. It may present itself in the song of a bird calling from a nearby tree or in the melodic vocalizations of whales we have overheard as we eavesdrop on their undersea conversations. Music may reach us through a radio or other electronic device, or it may be heard in what some describe poetically as the "music of the spheres."

Oliver Sacks describes another more personal and direct way in which music enters and informs our lives. In his descriptions of his own and others' experiences coping with neuropsychological injury, music appears as both an originator and companion of transforming experience. It is both agent and witness to the coherence of life.

At a climactic moment in the course of his recovery in the hospital from the injury he sustained to the muscles and nerves of his leg, Sacks speaks of a sudden encounter with a spiritual manifestation of music, as he experienced his body—his entire self—becoming re-integrated, in thought, in perception, and in action. Struggling to command his injured leg to move, to "get in step/get in tune" with the rest of his body in order to walk again, Sacks found the sounds and rhythms of Mendelssohn's Violin Concerto infusing his consciousness, coming to him through his body's memory. The sound of the music within him was fused with a spiritual experience he calls grace.

— *Suddenly—into the silence, the silent twittering of motionless frozen images—came music....Everything was transformed, absolutely, in that moment, in that leap from a cold fluttering and flashing to the warm stream of music, the stream of action, the stream of life...an organic whole...a unity....What appeared with the music was organization and center, and the organization and center of all action was an agency, an "I." What appeared in this moment transcended the physical, instantly orga-*

nized and reorganized it into a seamless perfect whole. This new, hyperphysical principle was Grace. Grace, unbidden, appeared on the scene, became its center, transformed the scene. Grace entered, at the very center of things, at its hidden innermost inaccessible center, and instantly coordinated, subordinated, all phenomena to itself. It made the next move obvious, certain, natural. Grace was the prerequisite and essence of all doing.

In his exploration of the intimate relationship between neurological, psychological, and spiritual injury and recovery, Sacks describes music as motivator and organizer, not just of voice or emotions but of nerve pathways, muscle fibers, and of the sensory integrative functions in the central nervous system. The sustaining and integrating function of music, he suggests, is as intrinsic to human life as is the electrical spark that keeps the heart beating.

The music that serves to kinesthetically organize, neurologically stimulate, and emotionally energize is different for each individual. During the course of her recovery from being struck by lightning, Gretel Ehrlich speaks of the roles of music in her efforts to heal as liberator, companion, and comforter. Music served also as a reminder and an echo of the rhythms of her body—walking, pulsing, moving across the earth—at a time when she could barely maintain consciousness long enough to stand and move across the room of her small cabin. The music of South African composer Kevin Volans was often her companion, reasserting the vital connections between her physical, emotional, and spiritual determination to live.

Joe Simpson would not have described the music that accompanied his agonizing hours of struggle on Siula Grande as helpful, sublime, or happy. Often music was a diversion or amusement for him as he remembered various tunes. There was one moment, however, when he experienced the steady drone of a remembered song that he hated—a song sung by a popular British rock group—as an assault on his conscious-

CHAPTER 4: ENERGIES TO SURVIVE

ness. Yet, I wonder if this remembered rhythm—insistent, loud, and obnoxious—echoed his body's fractured but determined insistence on living, despite the extremity of his physical injury and exhaustion. Perhaps Simpson was hearing his body's compromised heart rhythms, thrumming in loud and somewhat chaotic pulses, insisting on life, even when he was ready to collapse into exhaustion and death.

Similarly, Aron Ralston, the young climber who was trapped in a slot canyon in Utah for six days and who had to amputate his wrist to survive, noted in his hour-by-hour account of his survival experience that he had "the same song stuck in my head for forty-three hours." And it wasn't even "a real song," he exclaims in exasperation. It was a looping of sound with repeated letters and numbers, which infuriated and distracted him. He wonders, however, if perhaps the insistence of the music was keeping him from slipping into the sleep of hypothermia, the sleep of surrender to death.

Music seems to serve not only as organizer, motivator, comforter, and annoyer, it also can act as a sort of commander of the body's forces. Again turning to descriptions offered by Oliver Sacks, one finds further examples of the complex role that music can play in survival.

In his struggle to make his way down the mountain in Norway, with his leg damaged and dangling, sending loud messages of pain throughout his body, Sacks observes that "there came to my aid now melody, rhythm and music....I did not contrive this. It happened to me. I fell into a rhythm...." And in that rhythm his fear was subsumed and his body's resources marshaled to attention in order to continue his efforts to descend the mountain to safety.

At its most fundamental, music is the echo of the body's rhythm, the heart's rhythm, that declares "I am!" Music can take away, at least for a moment, the dread of panic, the submission to defeat, the surrender to danger, the comfort of unconsciousness, and fill the void of despair with its assertion of life.

Hope

When we talk about how a person is able to survive profoundly shattering injuries and suffering, whether caused by disease or terrible loss, accident, natural disaster, or violence, the question of hope is always present. In order to understand our own efforts and those that others have made to endure traumatic experience and its legacies, it is important to understand our ideas and attitudes concerning hope.

There is a general assumption that we all know and agree on what we mean when we use the word "hope." We assume that hope offers an optimistic view of one's situation or circumstances, suggesting a positive outcome. However, people who have endured diverse kinds of traumatic experiences tell us that hope does not have a single meaning. It is a complex experience, attitude, and viewpoint. For instance, many trauma survivors speak of experiencing "deceptive" or "false" hope, or "forlorn hope," and they warn that hope may or may not be a useful mental or emotional partner in time of need. Hope, they tell us, can be a trickster, appearing in many different guises: as tempter, cheerleader, messenger of bad advice, and also as wise counselor.

A young mountaineer named Art Davidson was one of the three climbers trapped at 18,200 feet above sea level for days, in clouds and snow and cold, on the face of Denali in Alaska, in January 1967. He describes the role of hope in the seduction of the traumatic process:

— *We continued to stare into the cloud, hoping it would break open to let us descend. Hoping—we had come to understand it so well that it had lost much of its meaning; but none of its appeal. I decided that to hope was to ignore the reality of our situation in favor of a wishful belief that some stroke of luck would befall us. No one could come for us through this whiteout. I berated myself for ever hoping, and warned myself never to hope again. Faith was what I lacked. I needed faith that this whiteout, like any stretch of foul weather, would eventually end; and faith that we'd have the presence of mind and stamina to take advantage of that moment when it came. I told Dave we'd be lost if we stopped believing in ourselves....Several minutes later I realized I was once again staring at the clouds, hoping they'd part.*

What is the relationship between hope and faith, between hope and belief? Art Davidson suggests that "believing in ourselves" is a necessity for survival and that hope is an unreliable but insistent and seductive tempter that may lead one into danger, not to safety.

Natan Sharansky also made strong distinctions between different kinds of hope and between belief and hope. As he struggled daily to cope with the effects of imprisonment in the Soviet gulag system, he reflected deeply on the essentials of survival. He saw that hope may be used to evade the reality of the moment. A person who lives on "false hope" can be weakened, Sharansky asserts. Hope can be an enemy to finding meaning and real strength in oneself. He writes:

— *In time I also understood what a cunning and deadly enemy even hope can be....If you don't see the meaning of the life you are leading this very minute, if it appears only when you live on the hope of rapid changes, then you are in constant danger.*

    If...life today seems meaningless, man inevitably makes himself see the end of it on a near horizon....But in the end, deceptive hope poisons the soul and weakens the spirit.

    During these years I have met people who have been weakened from constant disappointments. They continually create new hopes for themselves, and as a result they betray themselves. Others live in the world of illusions, hastily and incessantly building and rebuilding their world in order to prevent real life from ultimately destroying it.

> *What then is the solution? The only answer is to find the meaning of your current life. It's best if you are left with only one hope—the hope of remaining yourself no matter what happens. Don't fear, don't believe, and don't hope. Don't believe words from the outside; believe your own heart. Believe in that meaning which was revealed to you in this life, and hope that you will succeed in guarding it.*

Sharansky seems to suggest that it is the very personal and unique meaning of one's life that provides the essential "energy" of survival. This is a very different concept from hope. Or is it? If "meaning" is understood as an assertion of connectedness with beloved others or with a concept of greater good or with one's spiritual foundation or with the wholeness of oneself, then perhaps it is not so different from hope. For what is hope if not a bridge: a connection between the valued parts of oneself that extends backward into one's past, through the suffering of the present, and leads into the future? Hope may be thought of as a fragile thread: a bridge from the pain and dread, defeat and despair of traumatic experience, to a vision of wholeness and worth, dignity and self-determination.

Like Sharansky, Jerome Groopman, a physician and author, points out the pitfalls of "false hope," noting that it can lead to making poor medical decisions, which may compromise a person's health and ability to survive. The ability to hope, asserts Groopman, is dependent in part on neurochemical functions of the body, which can be disrupted by illness, deprivation, assault, or other physical conditions. As he explores the delicate interdependence of neurochemicals, thinking processes, and feeling states, in his book *The Anatomy of Hope*, Groopman gives examples of individuals who are able to maintain hope in the most extreme situations of medical disease. "It is part of the human spirit," he says, "to endure and give a miracle a chance to happen." If this is so, however, then why do

CHAPTER 4: ENERGIES TO SURVIVE

some people stop hoping and seem to give up, when medical facts would suggest they might be able to survive?

When a definition of hope is linked with the notion of "resilience," it might lead one to think that, despite hardships and even catastrophic events, hope will remain intact—apart from traumatic collapse—and help one to rise from the crush of defeat and loss. However, the facts don't bear out such a view. What the accounts of survivors of traumatic experience indicate is that hope may be extinguished in the face of "surrender to inevitable danger." The ability to hope is based on a subjective appraisal of one's circumstances and one's strengths. A person may understand, from a deep awareness of and connection with his or her own bodily processes, that to hope for recovery or rescue or "return to normal life" is a false hope. And it is important for others not to promote false hopes in the face of such a deeply personal appraisal.

Maintaining hope depends, also, on there being some connections remaining between parts of the self (feelings and thoughts, body and feelings, thoughts and body) and with at least the image of, if not the actual presence of, connection with other(s). If traumatic collapse has severed all of those connections, so that the structure or core of the self is entirely cut off, then hope is outside the grasp of the individual.

For this reason, it may become necessary at times for one to hold hope for others when they cannot hold onto it for themselves. As an example, a physician may understand that there is some hope for a person to survive, even though that patient may feel she has exhausted all of her resources to continue the struggle for life. Sometimes it is mainly through that single piece of connection—that hope held by the doctor or a beloved—that the small spark of life can be maintained and nourished.

As another example, I think of Joe Simpson lying in the snow among boulders, at the end of his strength. He called out for Simon, as if it were the very finish of his life, defiantly asserting his need for a witness to his utter aloneness. Simon responded—without thought, without reason—

based on the hope he carried that Joe would still be alive. As improbable as it seemed to him that Joe could be calling his name in the darkness, Simon responded, holding to that last fragile thread of connection between them.

CHAPTER 5

Principles, Plans, and Strategies

"Believe your own heart. Believe in that meaning which was revealed to you in this life."
—NATAN SHARANSKY

There is an "energy of life" that is beyond our control, beyond our conscious will to summon, which can—like magic—ignite a spark or fan a tiny ember of life and lead to a new opportunity to survive. There are desires deep within our bodies to keep life going, even though our reason would say it's time to quit. As well, thoughts and yearnings may drive our bodies to endure long beyond their expected capacities, enabling a miracle to take place.

Just as there are unconscious and often inexplicable internal resources that may come to our aid in times of trauma, we may experience also a sharpening of focus on conscious strategies and plans to get through the catastrophic events and circumstances we face. Such efforts are not generally "heroic" in and of themselves, in their scope or skills, though their end results may seem heroic indeed. Rather, such plans and strategies are often banal, common-sensical, the stuff of clichés. For instance, many survivors talk of the importance of "putting one foot in front of the other," of "keeping one's face pointed toward the sun," of "brushing one's teeth and combing one's hair each day," of "conserving energy," of "slamming shut the door" to thoughts of surrender or defeat. These are not fancy concepts: they are the real ingredients of endurance—of the effort to maintain oneself intact in the face of terrible loss.

As one listens to how these strategies have been implemented in times of extreme duress or catastrophe, it becomes clear that it is not the specific activity itself but the purpose it serves that is most important. The critical efforts one makes are directed to accomplish very basic functions—to find ways to remember and affirm the essential dignity of oneself, to maintain connection with others that reflects one's essential continuity and integrity, to preserve the ability to comfort oneself, and to find a safe place within oneself to retreat from the onslaught of suffering. Such functions do not necessarily assure continued life. They are directed, above all, toward affirming the basic meaning, or reason for being, of one's life, whether that physical life is able to continue into the future or not.

As I have listened to and read harrowing accounts of disaster and suffering, I have often thought that certainly I could not have managed such a terrible ordeal. When one thinks of enduring years in Auschwitz or of the relentless accretion of losses brought on by Lou Gehrig's disease or of crawling out of the chaos of an earthquake, it is hard to imagine that I have what it takes to endure. If I am expected to be a hero and to be strong or to keep my feelings under control, then—knowing me—certainly I shall fail miserably. Moreover, if I assume that I must remain alive in order to accomplish the goal of navigating traumatic experience successfully, then I may fail also.

But what if we are to understand that dying is not a defeat nor a sign of failure: that it is simply the natural consequence of the particular circumstances and processes in which we find ourselves at a particular time? What if there is really nothing more expected of me than to be myself, regardless of the outcome of the experience holding me in its grip—whether I am caught in a blizzard on a mountainside or held as a political prisoner; whether I am giving birth to a baby or witnessing the murder of

CHAPTER 5: PRINCIPLES, PLANS, AND STRATEGIES

a beloved; whether I have been struck by lightning or am trapped in an abusive family? To endure the hardships of traumatic experience, perhaps what is most needed is for a person to be his or her most "authentic self" (a phrase often used by Joseph Campbell). Out of the effort to remain most essentially oneself will then come the plans and strategies that are most specifically and uniquely suited to who I am and how I will act.

When Natan Sharansky describes the horrors of his nine years of imprisonment in the Soviet gulag system in his book *Fear No Evil*, the reader soon realizes that Sharansky's goal was not so much to stay alive, although he certainly wanted to live to see his family again and to emigrate to Israel to be with his wife. Instead, all of his efforts were directed toward implementing one simple principle, which he stated in the form of advice to others: "believe in that meaning which was revealed to you in this life, and hope that you will succeed in guarding it." The meaning that Sharansky found in his life, which only became clear to him when he was a young man in his twenties, was his deep rootedness in his Jewish heritage. The right and freedom to live out this heritage was denied him by the Soviet state; he was tried for treason and sent to prison for asserting that right publicly. The meaning of Sharansky's life was expressed also in his loyalty and devotion to his family and to his wife.

Oppression by the state, enacted relentlessly against Sharansky both outside and in the prisons where he was held for nine years, was the "evil" against which he struggled. The representatives of the oppression sought to tear apart his connections with his internal beliefs, along with his ability to feel and his ability to reason and make decisions. They also sought to isolate him from those people most dear to him. Against this assault Sharansky resisted openly, with integrity and strength.

The plans and strategies that grew from Sharansky's goal to maintain and guard the meaning of his life—his Jewish beliefs and heritage and their expression in his family and marriage—were also simple and straightforward. First, he refused to cooperate in any way with those people who sought to accuse him of wrong-doing—the KGB in particular—since the "wrong" of which he was accused was to practice his beliefs. He also refused to do or say anything that would bring harm to other political and religious activists and prisoners. All of his contacts with the KGB and authorities were based on his resistance to their version of the "truth," which distorted his true intentions and deepest moral convictions.

Second, Sharansky gave no power to his captors and guards. He treated them "like the weather." He explains: "I realized that nothing they did could humiliate me. I could only humiliate myself—by doing something I might later be ashamed of....I repeated this principle over and over until it was part of me: Nothing they do can humiliate me. I alone can humiliate myself."

In his relationships with other prisoners, Sharansky determined that he could best maintain his own integrity by treating all other prisoners with equal respect and even-handedness. He would not allow the system to manipulate him to turn against others. In this way he was able to maintain vital connections with others who shared the circumstances of his suffering, helping to decrease his isolation.

A fourth principle and strategy was to keep the small book of Psalms his wife Avital had given him by his side or in hand at all times. This book was not only the emblem of his faith and his heritage, but it also served as evidence of his enduring connection to Avital. In this way the "meaning in life" that defined his struggle had tangible form.

Finally, Sharansky insisted on the human right of connection to those he loved, through written communication and visits. His daily plans and strategies often served the purpose of resisting his captors' efforts to cut him off from all contact with his wife and family. (Avital had been able to emigrate to Israel just a day after they were married. She could not return to the Soviet Union to see her husband. Thus, she fought unceasingly from afar for his release and his right to emigrate.)

CHAPTER 5: PRINCIPLES, PLANS, AND STRATEGIES

Sharansky spent days and months in life-threatening hunger strikes to protest the KGB's withholding of letters and visits. If it meant that he must die to uphold this most important principle, Sharansky felt, then so be it. He would have preserved his integrity in the process.

In order to endure the consequences of his strategies, the reprisals from his captors, Sharansky describes very personal activities that helped him to calm his body and to regain a sense of personal control. One of his most enjoyable activities was playing chess—alone in his thoughts or with other prisoners, tapping the moves on pipes and walls. "Since childhood," Sharansky writes, "I have always used chess to escape from pressure and anxiety.... the game gave me power over grown-ups." Moreover, "the chess game was an attempt to impose order on my racing and chaotic mind...it provided a logical plan, was comforting and offered a sense of control."

Thus, to play chess, for Sharansky, was to reconnect with a part of his past in which he could regulate, to some degree, his levels of stress and into which he could bring himself comfort. Chess also helped him to maintain a sense of continuity in his life: that is, a reminder that he had a past and that the person he was in the past, though a child, was still the person he was in the present—a person who likes to play chess. In addition, he was able to use the game to be in contact with others, decreasing the lonely isolation of their separate cells.

Another activity in which he found comfort, particularly during the physical stress of his months-long hunger strikes, was a kind of relaxation exercise. In it he would systematically review his life, remembering details of family and friends and treasured activities with them. He could take himself out of the confines of prison and restore a sense of "normalcy" in what was the most abnormal of circumstances by retreating into this reverie. Because his relationship with Avital was his essential "anchor" to his meaningful life, such reveries—in which she played a very large role—carried him closer to himself and all that he cherished.

As mentioned earlier, Sharansky believed there is "an interconnection of human souls" that not only sustains us through dark times but to which we also have an obligation to conduct our lives with honor and moral integrity. This interconnection of souls transcends the limitations of time and space and circumstance and requires us to examine our own actions and principles in light of their reverberations throughout time.

Nelson Mandela's autobiographical account of his decades-long struggle against the oppression of apartheid, as told in his book *Long Walk to Freedom*, adds further dimensions to understanding how principles, plans, and strategies evolve in the course of profoundly distressing experiences. Mandela's ability to endure almost three decades in prison, fully a third of his life, and not be broken, not become vengeful, not lose hope nor his vision for his people, required deep strength, resolve, and integrity in the face of terrible hardships, degrading conditions, and constant threats. By his own account, his endurance, survival, and eventual victory over apartheid and oppression required Mandela to remain most truly and deeply himself. He explains:

> *We regarded the struggle in prison as a microcosm of the struggle as a whole. We would fight inside as we had fought outside. The racism and repression were the same; I would simply have to fight on different terms.*
>
> *Prison and the authorities conspire to rob each man of his dignity. In and of itself, that assured that I would survive, for any man or institution that tries to rob me of my dignity will lose because I will not part with it at any price or under any pressure. I never seriously considered the possibility that I would not emerge from prison one day.*

The deepest personal characteristics that Mandela identifies as those that helped him to endure are also those he identifies as belonging to all humans: dignity, generosity, and mercy. Thus, he appealed to those char-

CHAPTER 5: PRINCIPLES, PLANS, AND STRATEGIES

acteristics in the guards who watched over him and the officials with whom he negotiated for his release.

Mandela was in no way a passive man nor even "peaceful." His birth name was, in fact, "Troublemaker." He was willing to take up arms to fight against the oppression of the South African government, which created and codified the brutal policies of apartheid, and against the police who enforced them with violence. According to Mandela, active resistance does not negate but may in fact enhance the dignity and moral strength of oppressed people.

Nelson Mandela was born into leadership—his father was a Thembu tribal leader. He was schooled from the age of nine, when his father died, in the art and practice of democratic leadership in the home and councils of the acting regent of the Thembu people, a part of the Xhosa nation. For his entire life, Mandela has seen his own destiny inextricably linked to that of "his people," all of South Africans deprived of their human rights. He could not think of himself as a free man unless and until his people were free.

Throughout the years of his captivity, Mandela remained a leader: to other prisoners, to guards, and to the nation that heard his words of encouragement as they were carried out in smuggled messages and through the testimony of released prisoners. In the days and weeks he spent in solitary confinement, which he describes as the most difficult of all punishments to endure, Mandela held to the strength of his connection to his people, all those for whom he struggled, and thereby was able to withstand the terrors of isolation.

Over the years Mandela was able to bring small pieces of normalcy, even beauty, into the prison environment. He and other political prisoners taught each other courses in history, economics, and law. Through his prodigious powers of persuasion, he received permission from wardens and guards to grow a small garden of flowers and vegetables, which he shared with them and which enhanced their meager diets. Through continuous efforts large and small, he refused to yield to the desolation and brutality of those who kept him captive.

Imprisonment, Mandela writes, is "designed to break one's spirit and destroy one's resolve...to exploit every weakness, demolish every initiative, negate all signs of individuality—all with the idea of stamping out that spark that makes each of us human and each of us who we are." Mandela resisted such oppression, as Sharansky did, by affirming his absolute connection to those who struggled for the same cause: for freedom, for the right to pursue one's life with dignity, and for justice.

In a small, personal act, he affirmed also his hope for the future, by bestowing the name Zaziwe, or "Hope," on his daughter Zeni's first child. For the first time since he had been sent to prison, some fifteen years earlier, Mandela was able to embrace his daughter, and he was able to hold the new life she brought to him. In this act of ceremonial naming, he asserted his traditional role as grandfather and his unbreakable ties to his family. He also gave voice and name to his unquenchable optimism that justice would prevail over evil and that there would be a future of freedom for his grandchild.

For some of us, our sense of personal meaning may not seem as clear or well-defined as it was for Mandela or Sharansky. Not all of us feel so inextricably connected to a larger social or moral cause. In fact, for many of us, the "bottom line"—that which is most meaningful and worth fighting for in our lives—may only become clear when extreme circumstances force such an awareness into consciousness.

Remembering Beck Weathers, for instance, as he lay in a hypothermic coma on the upper reaches of Mt. Everest, left for dead, we understand from his own account that only in that most extreme situation did he come to realize his family held the deepest meaning for him in his life. Only when the images of his wife and son and daughter sprang to life before his eyes did he realize that he had to go to them. From that point

CHAPTER 5: PRINCIPLES, PLANS, AND STRATEGIES

forward, all of his plans and strategies served the purpose of moving him toward them.

This revelation takes on added significance when Weathers reveals that in his everyday life before this moment on the mountain he had consigned his family to a secondary role in his life and steadily resisted their efforts to draw him close. Yet at this moment of "death-in-life," Weathers knew with certainty that he had to make every effort to be with his family again. And so he rose out of the snow, chose a direction to walk down the mountain, woke from a coma a second time to ask for help, and defied all medical predictions to survive. His basic strategy consisted of "putting one foot in front of the other" and finding a way to get to help to return to his family.

The goal toward which Joe Simpson struggled and in the service of which he endured terrible suffering, was to resist—until the end of his strength and ability—surrendering to utter aloneness and abandonment, to trauma itself. Only as he reached the absolute limit of his endurance was he able to recognize that he could not bear the thought of dying alone— with no witness, with no one to take notice.

Such a revelation of personal need and meaning, of affirming his deep connection with others, stood in contrast to Simpson's persona as a member of the climbing world. Simpson has described himself, with no small amount of ironic humor, as a very stubborn person—stubborn not just in his determination to endure his ordeals on the formidable mountain Siula Grande but obstinate and provocative in the bars and on the streets of his hometown and in the familiar watering holes of the mountaineering community. This observation is corroborated in the Foreword to *Touching the Void*, in which Chris Bonington, a fellow mountaineer, candidly notes that Simpson was an "abrasive" sort of fellow. In addition, Richard, the young acquaintance who stayed at camp while Joe and Simon climbed Siula Grande, was frank in saying—on camera in the film—that Joe was hard to get along with. Compared to Simon, Richard said, Joe was the fellow you'd rather leave behind, if it came to that.

Yet it is this very stubbornness, this hard-edged, hard-driving, do-it-my-own-way personal characteristic that seemed to fuel Joe Simpson's unrelenting effort to get off the mountain and, finally, to reach camp. In Simpson's case, then, being his "authentic self" meant being a stubborn, hard-to-get-along-with guy, who would drive himself to reach his goal. It meant maintaining his daring, which in "normal" times would frustrate and frighten others, in order to make the necessary decisions that gave him a chance to survive. By being most completely himself Simpson came to that terrible choice to lower himself deeper into the crevasse in order to find a way out and to survive. Aron Ralston's decision to amputate his hand in order to save his life was consistent with his characteristic capacity to take on terrifying mountaineering objectives alone.

In contrast to Nelson Mandela, who was a "father" to his people and identified entirely with the cause of freedom for his entire nation, Joe Simpson was most authentically an individualist, a person who took pride in finding his own way in difficult circumstances. He was at home in the most remote mountains of the world and found pleasure in tackling impossible endeavors alone. Just as Mandela's identification with the larger community and cause framed his entire struggle to endure imprisonment, so did Simpson's self-reliant, individualistic orientation help him to endure. And at the end of his endurance Simpson found the understanding within himself that he needed the presence of a companion, another human soul, at his moment of extreme suffering.

Each Struggle Is Unique

Finding one's way in the face of the fragmentation and loss that defines traumatic experience requires both grace and fight. It is an opportunity to discern one's deepest meaning. It calls on music and muscle, focus and imagination, determination and reverie. There is no "right way" to endure the terrors and hardships of disaster, disease, or imprisonment. There is no one-size-fits-all spiritual path to withstand the horrors and isolation of suffering, pain, and grief. There is only the very personal struggle in the experience of each moment.

What is clear in this mysterious mix of mind, spirit, body, and desire is that each person's response to traumatic suffering and collapse is uniquely his or her own. By inquiring with an open mind and listening with all senses tuned to receive new perspectives, we can learn from each other what has transpired in each unique situation and how these insights might bring new understanding to our own lives.

Thinking back to descriptions and definitions of the traumatic process discussed in earlier chapters, we may now understand more fully that the efforts and activities of a person who seeks to endure the experience of trauma are most fundamentally efforts to maintain one's wholeness, autonomy, and self-regulation. Such goals are aimed at sustaining the most essential elements of what we think of as one's personhood—one's self. In some circumstances this may mean that death is the inevitable consequence; in others, it may mean that a person will form an alternate life, with the unbearable suffering encapsulated behind closed compartments in the mind and feelings. Or it may mean that pain and suffering become the activating and energizing forces for continued life. For many fortunate people, a new life may emerge in the wake of traumatic experience in which the trauma becomes a memory that does not intrude but informs and enriches. As we have said before, there is no "right way" to endure and resolve the traumatic process.

CHAPTER 6

Legacies: Transmission of Trauma

*"Perhaps we are like stones; our own history and the
history of the world embedded in us, we hold a sorrow deep within
and cannot weep until that history is sung."*
—SUSAN GRIFFIN

When my mother was a little girl of about eight years old, the family doctor told her that she had to go to the hospital because she had an infection in her leg. Her mother, my grandmother, took her there but soon was told to leave while nurses prepared my mother for surgery. What the little girl believed, as she lay alone on the hospital gurney, was that she was being prepared to die. She saw the stern and sorrowful-looking faces of the nurses; she had seen the worry in her mother's eyes before she left; she heard the doctor say it was very serious, indeed. And she could feel it: the infection—and the fear—were spreading throughout her body; there was hardly any room left to breathe.

When she became conscious again in the recovery room after the surgery, it took a long time for my mother to understand that she was still living. She had been so certain that she had come to the hospital to die.

Twelve years later, my mother rushed to the same hospital to give birth to her first child, my sister. No one had explained to her exactly what to expect in childbirth. She approached the event with a mixture of excitement and dread. She did not want to be in a hospital again. She held firmly to the conviction, throughout her life, that hospitals were where you go to die. This may reveal a subjective appraisal on my mother's part that she did, indeed, lose her life in some very significant sense in these traumatic experiences in the hospital. (I am reminded of Joe Simpson's poignant statement at the climax of his traumatic experience: "I lost me.")

Since my mother and my grandmother were of a generation and social group that did not permit the discussion of bodily functions, including childbirth, my mother entered her experience of giving birth with no real knowledge about how she had become pregnant, how a baby is born, or what to expect from her body, her emotions, or her caretakers during the childbirth experience. She did know, however, that her mother had suffered nerve damage during her own birth. Throughout the years my grandmother complained about the terrible pain she had experienced in childbirth. With each telling she seemed to blame my mother, her only child, for her suffering.

My father was prevented from being with his young wife during her hours of labor or in the delivery room. The doctor was late, so my mother's legs were tied together to prevent the baby from emerging until he finally arrived to deliver the baby. She was expected to give birth "naturally," so the administration of anaesthesia was delayed for many hours. It is clear from my mother's description that her pain and isolation and the uncertainties related to giving birth to her first child, were overwhelming for her—just as she had been overwhelmed as a little girl, alone in the same hospital.

The legacy of these traumatic experiences became a sort of code by which my mother lived her life, a code that insisted one must always be on guard and ready to ward off traumatic injury—that events may rise up at any time to take over your life and render you helpless, terrified, without words or means to defend yourself. She became, as an adult, a fearful,

CHAPTER 6: LEGACIES: TRANSMISSION OF TRAUMA

watchful woman, always on the lookout for that moment of "inevitable danger" in which she could be overwhelmed once again.

One of the tragic aspects of this legacy was that my mother felt she had to bear it in silence. How could she speak about something she could not understand or explain to herself? What words were there to tell others of the terror that had overtaken her life as a little girl and again as a young woman. There were no words adequate to tell her story, she concluded. It seemed uncertain to her, also, that there was anyone who would listen and understand her experiences.

My mother was haunted both day and night with the deeply felt but largely unconscious traces of the terrors that had assailed her early in her life. Although she spoke on occasion about frequent nightmares that intruded on her sleep, neither she nor her family and friends suspected their origin or understood their meaning as evidence of her past trauma. My mother's persistent anxiety and dread—frequently translated into physical pain—were expressed in many diffuse fears, often focused on the safety of my sister and me. However, if you were to ask my mother what frightened her or if she was sad or if past experiences bothered her, she would not be able to tell you and would dismiss your questions as silly. Her silence was like a rock. And that is what she called herself: the rock.

My mother sought relief from her constant terror and dread through a lifelong addictive reliance on prescription medications, alcohol, and cigarettes. Unfortunately, the chemicals only exacerbated her feelings of shame and helplessness and brought her little real respite from her emotional memories of pain and fear. Neither my sister nor I understood the connection between her persistent self-medication and her past traumatic experiences until a decade before her death.

Perhaps my father knew the depths of his wife's fears and loneliness, but he, too, was scarred by trauma. When he was a very young boy, my father's older brother died suddenly of an illness. Then, when my father was twelve, his father died unexpectedly of a heart attack. Like my mother, my father could not and would not talk about his feelings or past experiences. I never heard directly from him that these losses had occurred. He was firmly committed to sealing them off in the past. Because his early traumatic experiences related to sudden and devastating losses, first of his brother, then his father, it is not surprising that his major expression of such losses and grief was lifelong depression and migraine headaches. When such grief goes unspoken and unexplored, it must find expression somehow.

Like many others who have been injured by terrible life experiences, my mother took solace in poetry and great works of literature. She loved the poems of the 19th-century poet Lord Byron, especially *The Prisoner of Chillon*, a long narrative poem about a 16th-century political prisoner locked away in the dungeons of the Castle of Chillon on Lake Geneva. In this beautiful and haunting poem the full course of traumatic process is dramatized: suffering and grief are given a full voice.

I traveled with my mother one summer to the Chateau of Chillon, perched on the edge of Lake Geneva. Standing there in the dark, stone underworld prison, we witnessed the pathways made in the stone floor by the endless circling of the prisoner's footsteps four hundred years earlier, and we listened as another American visitor spontaneously recited many verses from Byron's famous poem. My mother was transported into the world of suffering evoked so powerfully by the poet, a world with which she wholeheartedly identified. Only a poet could provide the words adequate to express her own sorrows.

Many years later, when my mother was in her mid-seventies, I shared with her some of my thoughts and a series of graphic representations I had prepared for an upcoming presentation on trauma. My mother responded in an ordinary, matter-of-fact tone that what she had gone through in her young life was far worse than any of the stories or illustrations I had offered. I felt shocked to hear her say this. It was new and stunning to hear my mother say that anything had been amiss in her early life, much less to hear her use the word "trauma" to describe her own experiences.

CHAPTER 6: LEGACIES: TRANSMISSION OF TRAUMA

Quietly, I asked her what she was referring to and suggested we settle into comfortable chairs to talk. After more than fifty years of silence, my mother finally began to tell me her stories of traumatic experience for the first time. Unfortunately, a lifetime of resignation to pain and secrecy regarding her emotional life led her to dismiss her own stories as mere history and of no real significance to her any longer. No gentle prompting could encourage her to believe that I was truly interested in her experiences, past and present, nor could she trust that she would be understood. It was simply not safe, she believed, to reveal her feelings. Her continuing dread that the traumatic process would return to overwhelm her convinced her that she could never be safe.

For my sister and me, however, it was important to learn of my mother's experiences, even at this late date. Finally, there were real events to which we could attach the feelings of pain and panic, dread and isolation that had been floating freely among us in the family all these years with no anchor in facts, waiting for someone to claim them. At vulnerable times in our lives my sister and I had often found ourselves taking on these feelings as though they were our own, trying to resolve them in order to be free from them—a task that could not succeed, of course, since they didn't really belong to us.

The long-lasting effects of trauma experienced by my mother and our family are common to many people. The legacies of trauma shape and change people's lives in many and varied ways—and last for months, for years, or for a lifetime.

Transmission of Trauma

The silence that so often isolates people who have experienced trauma serves many purposes. Certainly its primary intention is to protect a person from further injury and suffering by refusing to give the memories of trauma reality by narrative communication. My mother's personal belief was, "If I don't talk about it, it didn't happen," a belief she voiced frequently, which was reinforced by our community's social contract that sought to deny distressing information through repressive social rules.

For others, silence is an expression of a fear that their stories of traumatic experiences might injure those they most want to protect: their children, family, and friends. And there is some justification for this concern about harming others with one's own traumatic experience; trauma can be "catching."

The "contagion effect" of trauma is a form of transmitting traumatic experience from one person to another that is so common in everyday life that we seldom take notice of it directly. It refers to the impact of visual, verbal, and auditory images of traumatic events that are communicated so successfully that other people experience the trauma as their own. For instance, in group settings where members who have experienced trauma have free rein to tell their stories in as much detail as they choose, other members of the group may find themselves feeling traumatized also, as though the experience belonged to them. Some people are particularly vulnerable to "catching" the distress of other people's experiences and making it their own because of their own history of trauma, whether recent or in the past. The impact of combining the distress communicated by another with one's own memories of suffering can become overwhelming.

Lenore Terr, a psychiatrist specializing in trauma, provides fascinating examples of famous writers, filmmakers, and poets, such as Stephen King, Alfred Hitchcock, and Edgar Allan Poe, who have recreated their own childhood trauma in such vivid and compelling artistic forms that their audiences are drawn into their stories and experience them with direct immediacy. (One needs only to remember the shower scene from the Alfred Hitchcock movie *Psycho* for an example of this effect, although this particular scene is not based on a childhood memory of a traumatic experience.) The entire traumatic experience is communicated, portraying the event itself and the feelings that accompanied the event, including dread, terror, and pain. The result is that the viewer, or reader, may feel that they have been traumatized by that specific event and may have fears related to similar events in the future (such as an aversion to taking a shower in a motel room).

In pioneering research, Terr also studied the direct aftereffects of trauma evidenced in the children of Chowchilla, CA, who were kidnapped and buried for days in their school bus. Her results provided compelling examples of ways in which children may transmit trauma to their playmates by recreating traumatic experiences in their games and play activities. Although all of the kidnapped children survived without physical injury, this single-event trauma had long-lasting, disrupting emotional effects on their lives and on their families and community.

Terr was able to observe that younger children, who had lived through the kidnapping, created games (which they called "school bus") enacting the story of their terrifying experience. Parents of children who had not been a part of the original kidnapping reported to Terr that these "innocent" children were terrorized, in turn, by their participation in the re-enacting games. From this and further observations of children who had been traumatized, Terr concluded that this type of re-enactment through play did not help the children master their feelings but served only to keep their fears active and spread them to others.

Another form of transmitting trauma, referred to as "the intergenerational transmission of trauma," works in a different way. Generally, this phenomenon results from the splitting apart of the emotional, rational, and physical parts of a traumatic experience from the events to which they belong. Each part then takes on a life of its own without reference to the specific events to which it is connected. These disconnected parts then dominate the personal interactions with family and friends.

For instance, my mother's feelings of terror, panic, and dread that belonged to her traumatic experiences of childhood surgery and of childbirth, were communicated forcefully and consistently to her family in myriad ways. However, the feelings did not correspond to any information she shared about her life. Quite the opposite: she painted a picture of her childhood and young adulthood as idyllic and denied distress throughout her life. Because children naturally identify with their parents and learn about feelings from them, my sister and I took as our own my mother's feelings of fear, but we didn't know their causes. Thus, we carried the feelings of a traumatic experience without having lived the experience itself. Similarly, one can receive other aftereffects of traumatic experience, such as emotional numbness, without being aware of what it is related to.

The far-reaching consequences of the inter-generational transmission of trauma have been greatly underestimated. This legacy affects not only individuals and families but also entire generations of people who are the children and grandchildren of those who have suffered communal traumas such as war or natural disaster. It has become clear in the sixty years since the end of the Second World War that many of the soldiers returning home shared a brotherhood of silence about their horrific experiences in war. This didn't preclude the aftereffects of their traumatic experiences from being transmitted to their families, however, through their rages, their disturbed sleep patterns, and their altered personalities. The soldiers' families, especially the children, received these emotional aftereffects of trauma as though they belonged to present family life rather than to past events. With no acknowledged events to explain this new array of feelings set loose in the family, it seemed logical to the wives and children to think that they had somehow caused them or were responsible for them. In this way the "war zone" was continued in the life of the family.

The Power of Silence

In his life's work of writing and speaking about the experiences and legacies of the Holocaust, Elie Wiesel suggests that giving voice to trau-

CHAPTER 6: LEGACIES: TRANSMISSION OF TRAUMA

matic experience provides a way to repair the splitting off of feelings from the facts of trauma—a way to give the experiences wholeness and reality. He exhorts survivors to tell their stories so that they and others cannot deny or be tempted to repeat the horrors they experienced and to which they bore witness. He believes that breaking the barrier of silence will assist not only the survivors but also their families and the larger society in which they live.

But Wiesel acknowledges also the difficulties that are inherent in remembering and speaking out about tragedies of such magnitude as war and genocide. When he and other survivors of the Holocaust tried to write the stories of their experiences, in an effort to honor the loss of their families and friends, they could find no language to describe what they had witnessed in the death camps. Moreover, when they tried to report what they had seen and experienced, they found that "people around us refused to listen; and even those who listened refused to believe; and even those who believed could not comprehend. Of course they could not. Nobody could. The experience of the camps defies comprehension."

I found myself thinking of Elie Wiesel's descriptions of the difficulties and tensions associated with speaking about traumatic experience when, quite by accident, I overheard two people of my parents' generation talking about whether or not to tell their own stories to their children.

This intensely personal conversation arose between a man and a woman who were sitting just a few feet away from me in the waiting room of a car repair shop. I was perusing the morning newspaper when they came in separately to the quiet, comfortable lounge area. Clearly they did not know each other. We were all strangers to one another.

Some small exchange of pleasantries began between the man and the woman. They seemed to be in their seventies, both tall, sitting with upright postures and with heads held high. The man had a courtly appearance. The woman's light brown hair was softened with silver and swept back elegantly from her strong, square face. Her soft voice carried traces of an accent belonging to another language, spoken in a different place long ago in her lifetime.

So quickly that I felt myself go very still, the conversation left the ordinary and became a story of revelation and drama. A shorthand of expression took form in which this man and woman spoke about shared tragedy of the past—each in their own countries, each with their own families, each in their own solitary darkness, yet nevertheless shared and known to the other.

All that remains in my memory of their conversation are these fragments and the long, full silences that were exchanged between them:

She: "But they can't understand what it was like then."

He: "No, but they seem to want to know."

She: "It was so hard. We had nothing. How can they understand that now?"

He: "I never wanted to think about it or talk about it. Now, I'm not sure."

She: "There was nothing. We lost everything."

He: "They seem to really want to know. My children gave me a tape recorder. They said to try to talk into it. They said they want to know what it was like."

She: "I couldn't do that."

He: "Well, I tried it a little. Actually it felt better to tell about it a little."

She: "I could never speak about it."

He: "You might try. It's really not too bad. And I think they do want to know."

What were these people talking about? I dared not move or make a noise for fear they would remember they weren't alone in this little room and would stop talking. Never did they reveal what their separate pasts held that was so fearful to remember and talk about. No specifics were

CHAPTER 6: LEGACIES: TRANSMISSION OF TRAUMA

mentioned that would give me, an outsider, a clue to their hidden memories. Yet it was certain they understood each other very well. In my imagination I thought of the Great Depression, of wars, and of the Holocaust—times of hardship, terrible loss, and deprivations. Any of these events were within the time span of their lives.

What remains for me the most vivid and poignant aspect of this scene was the great tenderness of the man toward the woman. His compassion was complete. He understood that she was alone with her memories, burdened by them, still suffering from them, and that she was fearful that the telling would harm her and those whom she told. He understood all this, and he offered her his own experience as an outstretched hand: he had tried talking about it, a little, and it was good. It was safe, he was saying, for her to try also, to tell her story.

The dilemma lived out in the conversation of this man and woman is one shared by a generation of trauma survivors. Elie Wiesel explains:

— *They have lived in isolation for a long time, locked away, remaining aloof so as not to wound those close to them. Whenever there was talk of the war years, they would clench their teeth and change the subject. It was impossible to get them to let go, to touch wounds that would never heal. They had reasons to be suspicious, to think that no one was interested in what they had to say, and that in any case they would not be understood....I shared with them my conviction that it is incumbent upon the survivors not only to remember every detail but to record it, even the silence. I urged them to celebrate the memory of silence, but to reject the silence of memory.*

For me survivors constitute a family like no other, an endangered species. We understand one another intuitively. We are haunted by the same past, the same problems concern us, the same mission moves us.

Survivors are a community of people, many of whom are trapped in silence: not just the survivors of the Holocaust but survivors like my mother. My mother was unaware that she was part of a larger group of women who also had experienced trauma in giving birth. None knew each other because they could not talk about their experiences; and so, like my mother, they remain isolated. The sense of being a part of a "family of survivors" only comes when the silence is lifted.

In some circumstances, silence is a passive response to traumatic suffering, one born of resignation to seemingly impossible alternatives. Not uncommonly, however, silence can serve as an active form of communicating profound injury. When words fail entirely and neither the survivor nor those around him can comprehend the enormity of the suffering that has occurred, silence may express more boldly what words cannot.

The active role of silence is well illustrated in the story of childhood trauma sustained by the poet, writer, and teacher, Maya Angelou, which she narrates in her book *I Know Why the Caged Bird Sings*.

When she was eight years old, Maya Angelou was raped. After the man who raped her was tried, sentenced to a year in jail, and then brutally murdered after his release, Angelou became mute for almost five years. She explains that her "silence was the only language" with which she could respond to these events.

Because she was a child, Angelou had no words with which to explain to herself or others the complicated story of what the man had done to her: not just the rape but the years before in which he had groomed her for his sexual abuses. Trying to reason out the experience of rape and murder within the framework of the deeply Christian teachings of her family, Angelou concluded that she was at fault. She linked her testimony in court to the death of the rapist. She was, therefore, evil. If she talked to anyone, she believed "that person might die too. Just my breath, carrying my words out, might poison people and they'd curl up and die…I had to stop talking…." Occasionally she talked to her beloved brother Bailey, the one person whom she knew understood her and the traumatic experiences of their childhood. With others she remained mute.

Ironically, this self-imposed exile into silence permitted Angelou to begin a long and intimate acquaintance with great writers, whose works she devoured. Even as a child, Angelou understood intuitively the "interconnection of human souls" that was offered to her by poets and writers—connections that would enable her to transmute her suffering and silence into kinship with them and an opportunity to form a new life.

A Need to Tell the Story

Silence stands at one end of a continuum of responses to traumatic experience that have a profound impact on the most basic aspect of human relationships: communication. At the other end of the continuum is a compelling need to tell—with words, in music, by painting and sculpture—the story of trauma: not once, but over and over. The profound need to tell and re-tell the story of trauma is a common, usually short-term aftereffect or legacy of traumatic experience. When it persists and is maintained as an effort to resolve the experience itself, it seldom succeeds.

The repetitive expression of traumatic experience often begins as an attempt to explore the event itself, in all of its detail: to become acquainted with an experience that could not be fully recognized or acknowledged as it occurred. At later times the repetition appears to be an effort to assert, by the act of giving it form, that there is meaning to the traumatic experience. Another objective to giving trauma expression is to bring the storyteller, musician, or artist into the company of others, with the hope of decreasing the isolating effects of the trauma.

Some or all of these reasons for expressing traumatic experience may drive a person to create various ways to communicate all or part of the story. The more successful the means of communication, the more the "audience" will "get the message." This may have the unintended effect of driving the audience away, causing people to reject the expression of traumatic experience for fear they might "catch" it themselves.

Surely the Norwegian artist Edvard Munch could not have anticipated the response he received when he first exhibited his painting *The Scream* (first titled *Despair*). He found himself and his painting the subject of public ridicule. Gallery patrons laughed in derision, and the artwork was discounted as foolish. It is likely the viewers' reactions did not derive so much from the expressionist techniques Munch used in his artwork but from the public's discomfort in witnessing such a bold depiction of terror and pain.

This makes all the more poignant Munch's 1892–93 description of the origins of this painting in which he wrote:

> *— I was walking along the road with two of my friends. Then the sun set. Suddenly the sky became bloody red, and I felt a tinge of melancholy, a sucking pain beneath my heart. I stopped, leaned against the railing, dead tired. Over the blue-black fjord and city hung blood and tongues of fire. My friends walked on and I stood again trembling with fright. And I felt as if a loud, unending scream were piercing nature.*

In a more succinct description, compiled by Munch in the 1930s, he wrote: "I walked along the road. With two friends as the sun set. The sky suddenly turned into blood and I felt the great scream in nature."

Munch's literal description of events signals to me that this is a picture of traumatic experience. The sky *turned into* blood. It did not look to him like blood; *it was blood*. The painting was a direct representation of experience, one that was utterly horrific and debilitating to him. Also of importance is that Munch suggests that the traumatic injury is not only to the man on the bridge, Munch himself, who feels a "sucking pain" and who "trembles with fright"—but also to nature: the sky bleeds, and a

CHAPTER 6: LEGACIES: TRANSMISSION OF TRAUMA

"scream in nature" is felt by the man. A wounded man and wounded nature: the two inseparably suffering.

What occasioned this experience (or perhaps it was a memory of traumatic experience?) is not known, and is subject to conjecture only. It is known that a distant volcanic eruption occurred at about the time when Munch noted the blood red color of the sky. Perhaps volcanic ash reflected the fiery flames of refracted light. Whatever the cause, the impact on Munch aroused deep emotions that are clearly shown in his painting.

Munch sketched and painted *The Scream* over and over, in many versions, all with the same intensity and expression of helpless horror and pain. Today this same image is copied again and again, and it is represented on familiar objects, such as coffee mugs. It has become a culturally accepted shorthand allusion to traumatic experience and an expression of a communal need to transform suffering, to tame it. The image of terror is rendered impotent, unable to cause pain to others, by placing it on a toy, a T-shirt, or household item. It is curious, however, that the image is treasured, nonetheless. We don't want to forget trauma altogether, only the frightening feelings that accompany it.

Did sketching and painting many versions of *The Scream* help Munch to resolve the traumatic experience(s) to which it referred? I'm not aware of any biographical material that would suggest an answer. The mere repetition of traumatic material, whether in literature, art, or music, is often as unproductive for adults as it was for the Chowchilla children who re-enacted their fears in games. Only when such compulsive repetition is accompanied by personal insight and is responded to with empathy, compassion, and understanding can it begin to yield relief and some resolution of the suffering that brought it to life.

CHAPTER 7

Legacies: The Brain, the Will, and the Body

"There was a lesion...in me."
—OLIVER SACKS

The long-lasting aftereffects of traumatic wounding take unique forms, all of which give proof of the severe and often debilitating disruptions of connections caused by the fragmentation of traumatic experience. The disruptions are internal as well as external. They cause a person to lose confidence in him- or herself as well as in others. Dread and terror can cause a person to retreat into silent suffering that may last for years or for a lifetime. Families and even generations can unwittingly take on as their own the feelings of fear and of self-blame that more correctly belong to the wounded member or group that has endured unspeakable horrors and injuries. Hypervigilance and hyperarousal, conditions of perpetual physical and emotional readiness to fend off disaster, exhaust the power to reason. These are only a few of the legacies of trauma.

Stories of trauma are seldom told in perfectly factual detail. When the body is roused into a state of vigilance, the neurochemicals that ensure a readiness to respond to danger influence how one perceives the "reality" of one's situation. Only after the danger is in the past and the body's chemistry has an opportunity to return to normal, can such perceptions be sorted through and understood.

Even then, however, long after external safety has been gained and life has resumed its normal pace, some individuals who have been profoundly injured by traumatic experience may continue to recall details of their experience in an altered form, drawn in the imagination like a piece of art that includes wishes and fears that cannot be permitted into conscious awareness.

This was the case for one of the older children who had been kidnapped and buried in the school bus in Chowchilla (as described by Lenore Terr). Many years after the event, the young man continued to give a narrative account of his own and the other children's escape from their buried bus which did not match, in some of its details, the "reality" of what he first saw when he emerged from the roof of the bus. He maintained steadfastly, however, that his account was "true." And for him it was.

I have come to understand from such accounts that if we insist on accuracy in narrative expressions of traumatic experience, we may miss an opportunity to understand the larger meaning of stories. Often, in the very details that seem "wrong" reside important clues that lead to a better understanding of the emotional significance to the survivor of the traumatic event.

Hypervigilance is one of the direct aftereffects of trauma that can become a disturbing legacy when it is not understood and cared for. It is one of the nervous system's primary responses to danger: a primitive, essential somatic activity that prepares us to avoid injury. Driven by the deepest level of our brain's function, this watchfulness or hyperalertness is largely out of our conscious control. When it persists over time, lingering long after its usefulness has passed in response to a frightening or traumatic event, it sometimes can be tempered, modulated, or transformed so as

CHAPTER 7: LEGACIES: THE BRAIN, THE WILL, AND THE BODY

not to interfere in daily life. For some who have suffered repeated, persistent danger, it may never be extinguished. A simple example of the useful aspect of hypervigilance is illustrated in the following scene.

A group of campers find themselves roused out of sleep by a grizzly bear that has come to ransack their food supply. Since these bear have been known to attack people, not just steal food, the campers have reason to be afraid and to seek safety by fleeing into the woods. Having helped itself to their tasty food, the bear leaves also. When the campers come back to their tents, they are on full alert for any signs of the bear returning. They are watchful: every sound in the brush makes them jump. They are ready to run. They are unable to sleep. And they tell and re-tell the story of the bear to each other. Its size, its sounds, even its intentions are perceived differently by each camper. They can all agree on one thing, however: they are fearful the bear will return and harm them. They must be extra vigilant.

Watch Out for Snipers

The following vignette describes a real set of events that affected a young woman whom I saw for consultation in my private psychotherapy practice some years ago. It serves to illustrate the way in which a survivor's story can be shaped by the powerful influence of hypervigilance to communicate important information about her traumatic experience.

When I first met Jan, her life had recently been threatened in a violent physical attack by a relative. It was a surprise attack, unlooked for and unprovoked. The assault was terrifying and humiliating; it threatened the balance of family relationships. The emotional and somatic aftereffects compromised Jan's stability and her physical health. Her intense fear, her shame at not being able to defend herself, and her worries about her children's and her own safety persisted for weeks and months after the event.

One day, about a month after the original assault, Jan came to my office with her husband, a quiet, earnest man who sought to understand his wife's feelings but who had not before faced such complex and profound psychological phenomena. As they arrived, it quickly became apparent that Jan was very agitated and frightened.

Once they were settled safely in my consultation room, Jan began to chastise her husband for being late to pick her up at her office to come to this appointment. Clearly her level of distress far outreached the immediate circumstances. They had, in fact, been only about five minutes late to the appointment. We were puzzled.

Finally, the full story emerged. Jan described to us how she had stood alone on the sidewalk outside her office building, located on a busy downtown street, waiting for her husband to come with the car, as they had planned. As she waited, she became increasingly worried and fearful, feeling entirely alone and isolated in a sea of strangers.

Suddenly she saw figures on a nearby rooftop. They were snipers, she said, aiming their weapons at her. She became terrified and felt there was no place to hide to avoid being wounded or killed. She felt paralyzed. Only when her husband's car pulled up beside her could she flee to safety. She had remained mute until she arrived at my office, where finally she felt safe enough to tell this story.

Just as it would have been disrespectful and of no benefit to question Edvard Munch's perception that "the sky suddenly turned into blood" or to insist that the boy who had been kidnapped had got some of his facts wrong, so it would have been ill-advised to question Jan's perception that there were snipers on the rooftops of our city. I have learned that such information must be understood as "real" in the language of trauma. It must be accepted and valued as a pathway to understanding the experience of traumatic wounding, which has no means to convey adequately its darkness, its loneliness, its terrible pain, and its desire for relief. Through her continued hypervigilance, Jan's nervous system sought to keep her

CHAPTER 7: LEGACIES: THE BRAIN, THE WILL, AND THE BODY

safe from further surprise attacks. Such intense, long-lasting watchfulness took a toll on her physical stamina and on her emotional equilibrium, however.

Fortunately, Jan's husband was able to understand the message the sniper scene provided: that of the profound nature of his wife's injury and its legacy of terror and hypervigilance. He understood her sense of vulnerability, and he offered her comfort in response. Until her actual safety from the person who had assaulted her was assured, however, she would not rest. She would remain on guard.

It is exhausting to live on the edge of panic all day and all night. It is debilitating to experience the sort of waking illusions that Jan did when she saw snipers. Adding to the terror she already felt when she remembered the assault on her life, she then had the horror of her own body and imagination creating images and feelings over which she had no control. Her loss of ability to calm herself and to lessen or modulate her fear added to her state of confusion, frustration, and grief. She no longer had "her life."

The hypervigilance that dominated Jan's life after she was attacked provides an example of the way in which normal psychophysiological functions can be activated in response to a traumatic event and then cannot be shut off after the event is over. In a life not affected by trauma, the self-regulatory functions of the body restore balance to the overall system after a particular need has passed. If a car horn honks as we start to cross the road, we feel a little jolt of adrenaline, step quickly back to the curb, and soon make the crossing without another thought about the changes that have taken place in our bodies and our perceptions to accommodate the demands of each moment.

In the aftermath of traumatic experience, the ability to self-regulate feelings, thoughts, and neurochemical responses is profoundly disturbed. What once was a "normal" capability or behavior can no longer be counted on. Vital connections are lost between parts of the self. The lines of communication between thinking and doing, feeling and reason, belief and desire are twisted, frayed, and sometimes severed.

When Feelings Have No Words

When feelings become disconnected from the words to name them, as a result of traumatic experience, the condition is called alexithymia. Others have called the experience one of "speechless terror." Without the assistance of language and symbol to describe and delimit the emotions of trauma, a sense of loss and confusion results.

A middle-aged woman came to my office some years ago with a simple request: "I want my feelings back," she said. She believed she had become separated from them in a past she could not remember as being remarkable. Now she was unable to know *if* she felt or what she felt. I must confess that at that time I really didn't understand fully what she meant, but I agreed to learn from her what it was that was amiss and to try to find a way to meet her wishes for help.

This articulate woman appeared to be a very normal, average person with many skills and strengths. She was well-educated, and—by all accounts—a successful wife and mother of three well-functioning, grown children. However, as we talked during the next many months, I learned that her early history was filled with incidents of sexual abuse that had been perpetrated by a relative who had also abused almost every member of her immediate and extended family. I came to understand that this was an entire realm of emotional experience for which she had no words. She could relate the facts of the horrific incidents of sexual abuse that she and other children in her family had experienced, yet she possessed no words with which to connect the facts with feelings that accompanied the abuse. Without words, the feelings themselves were inaccessible to her.

CHAPTER 7: LEGACIES: THE BRAIN, THE WILL, AND THE BODY

One day, after we had been meeting for many months, she told me a story of a particularly sad event that had occurred in her childhood. I noticed tears falling down her cheeks. Seeing me notice the tears, she took notice herself and put a hand to her cheek. Immediately she appeared bewildered and confused. She was quiet for some time and then asked: "What are these?"

I replied: "They are tears." She seemed at a loss to understand what was happening to her.

I ventured: "Those are tears, and you are crying because you are sad. What you have been telling me just now is very sad."

I paused and then continued: "In the past, when you experienced this injury to you, you were sad. It wasn't safe to show your feelings then; you had to pretend they weren't there. Now you are safe, and you feel sad today thinking about what happened to you and remembering how you felt then."

She was silent for a long time. Then she said: "These are my feelings. I'm feeling sad. I'm crying because I'm sad." She sighed and relaxed; she rested; and then she began to smile. "At last," she said, "I'm getting my feelings back."

The legacy of lost connections that had been in place for over forty years in the life of this woman could have retained its grip on her for an entire lifetime if other family members had not begun to reveal the long-held secrets of their own abuse. Only then were her own memories roused from hiding. Only then did she become aware of the missing pieces of her emotional life that had been effectively stored away for so many years.

Sometimes a person is forced to remember early experiences of trauma by hearing the stories of others who were also involved. Or anniversary dates may stimulate memories of the day a beloved child or husband or parent died or when the earthquake or lightning strike happened. Even as simple a fact as one's child becoming the age at which one's own traumatic experience occurred can trigger an unlooked-for onslaught of memories. Keeping memories at bay is not any easy task. Living with the legacies of traumatic injury may be even more difficult. Keeping the memory of trauma separate from everyday life requires a person to accept himself as less than whole, as less than the person he knows himself to be.

Cognitive Constriction

Laura, another middle-aged woman I counseled in a group for women who had been sexually abused in childhood, had come to think of herself as "dumb." As she began to remember and talk openly about her history of childhood abuse, she also began yearning to pick up threads of her life that had been dropped in the aftermath of her injuries. Laura understood intuitively that her self-perception of being "dumb" was attached to her past—was part of her response to trauma. Her decision to enter college at the age of forty-three, fulfilling a wish she had held silently for many years, took great courage. Despite her fears that she would be proved stupid—unfit for higher learning—Laura reported to the group, over a period of two years, that she was, in fact, an "A" student. Much to her relief and delight, she enjoyed college and was respected for her abilities.

I suspect that two main factors contributed to Laura's self-image of being dumb. The first was the impact of the experience of sexual abuse on her self-esteem. Often children blame themselves for abuses (or other traumatic events) that have occurred, believing that if they had been "smart enough" they could have avoided their injuries. They call themselves "dumb" and "stupid" in a regular litany of self-deprecation.

The second, less widely acknowledged factor that may have been at work to produce Laura's belief that she was too dumb to learn is the phenomenon of cognitive constriction, a direct aftereffect of trauma that can persist for a long time and contribute to a false assessment of a survivor's skills and capabilities. Simply stated, cognitive constriction is the narrowing of focus and mental activity that derives from the body's response to a

CHAPTER 7: LEGACIES: THE BRAIN, THE WILL, AND THE BODY

severe shock to its organization and structure. It is descriptively analogous, perhaps, to the shutting down of certain peripheral functions that take place in the process of hypothermia, as described earlier.

Although it might seem that cognition, or thinking, is a function critical to survival, it is not a core function such as keeping the heart beating, keeping oxygen flowing into the brain, and other such essential, involuntary activities that the body requires to maintain life. Thinking is a luxury in such circumstances. This narrowing of the field of attention and of reason is evidenced in the difficulties many people experience as they enter and exit the vortex of traumatic experience. Ordinary activities such as making simple calculations, finding one's way to a familiar place, paying attention, remembering names or dates, and a host of other tasks on which one depends to navigate everyday life become difficult or impossible to accomplish, both during and long after the traumatic event. It is very frightening to feel cut off in this way from one's own capacities to function, whether one is climbing Mt. Everest, recovering in a hospital from broken limbs, or coping with the return of memories of abuse and violence. A fearful question naturally arises: Will I be like this forever?

One day, some years ago, as I was attempting to describe to an audience of colleagues the utter frustration and feeling of helplessness engendered by cognitive constriction, a man who identified himself as a mental health professional interrupted my talk to challenge my sympathetic portrayal of the havoc that this disruption of mental functioning can cause. He asserted, somewhat dismissively, that all that is necessary to deal with cognitive constriction is to instruct "the patient" to make lists. One should set out problems and tasks in the form of lists, he said—lists of things to do, places to go, directions to get there, names of people to see—and all would soon be well again.

I admit to feeling quite baffled as to how I could reply to this man. What words could I use to impress on him that when traumatic experience tears apart the basic connections on which the integrity of the self is based, it is not a matter of list-making, or of willpower that can transcend such fragmentation?

In the silence that followed the man's assertions and my search for a useful response came the quiet, hesitant voice of a woman, reaching out from a dark corner in the back of the room. I could not see her; she was hidden in the shadows. Very softly she introduced herself as a professional woman, with several advanced academic degrees, who held a position of great responsibility and stature in the local healthcare field. In a direct and forthright manner she told the story of how, a few years earlier, unexpectedly she had recovered memories from her early childhood in which she had been the victim of severe physical abuse. She had been able to set aside an awareness of those experiences for over thirty years in order to complete the tasks of growing up and of making her way in life to fulfill her dreams for education, work, and family.

However, the flood of memories of those early childhood experiences had ruptured the walls that had contained them, and the rush of feelings, images, and thoughts attached to the memories overtook her and consumed her life. She lost her ability to take care of herself. She lost track of time and place. Her world became chaotic. For many months she could not work. She could neither be close to her husband nor care for her children. She described the experience of knowing what tasks she needed to do—to make lunch for the children, for instance—but she was entirely unable to carry out those ordinary activities. She no longer knew how to make lunch for the children. It was not a question of will. It was simply an impossibility.

She ended her brief comments by telling the hushed audience that it had taken her many months to regain even basic functioning. And now, some two years later, she was just beginning to feel confident that she could construct a new and full life that recognized her past and looked forward to a future. Only now could she find and count on the essential

CHAPTER 7: LEGACIES: THE BRAIN, THE WILL, AND THE BODY

connections between her thoughts, her wishes, her feelings, and her actions.

Willpower

In the aftermath of his fall on the mountain in Norway, Oliver Sacks experienced many ways in which the vital connections between the injured part of his body (his leg and what he wanted to do with it) had become entirely severed from his functional control. He could no longer experience his leg as being a part of himself, nor could he command it to move—or not to move. His hospital physicians, like the man who talked about making lists, were dismissive of Sacks' complaint of having "lost" his leg. Such a concept made no sense to the surgeon, who insisted that Sacks was "fine" and that he should be entirely able to perceive and control the functions of his leg. The implication was that Sacks was "malingering"—making up an incapacity that really didn't exist. For the wounded neurologist, this was indeed an insult to his self-concept that was already wounded by the utter helplessness encountered in his struggle to survive on the mountain and subsequently by the fact of his surgery and isolation in the hospital.

What was wrong, then? If his body had been repaired so that physiologically and neurologically all of the connections had been reattached, why couldn't he move his leg, even from one side of the bed to the other? Or why did his leg fall off the bed without his awareness, so that an angry nurse chastised him for "allowing" such a stupid thing to happen? Only in retrospect, after his body and his psyche had sufficiently healed from the trauma of his injury and as he studied more fully the phenomena of his traumatic experience, could Sacks put the pieces of this puzzle together. He writes: "All willing is willing *something*, and it was precisely that something which was missing…it was precisely this 'how,' the very idea, which was missing.…"

Sacks suggests that the injury he sustained could not be comprehended in purely physiological terms. It required a psychological and metaphysical understanding also. The tear to the muscles and nerves of his leg created a tear in his understanding of reality and of his place in that reality. He explains: "There was a breakdown of memory, of thinking, of will—not just a lesion in my muscle, but a lesion in me."

Sacks' pivotal concept, which emphasizes the psychophysiological nature of his traumatic wounding, provides a valuable clue to understanding other, diverse experiences of lost internal connections. For instance, the "breakdown of memory," the "lesion" in the self, articulated by Sacks, is descriptive also of core aspects of traumatic grief. What begins as a psychological wound or assault on the self becomes expressed in physiological forms, including neurasthenia and loss of affective expression, such as the inability to smile.

The fictional character, Sol Nazerman, who is central to the film and the novel *The Pawnbroker*, springs to mind as an example. I believe his character is so powerful and so memorable not only because of the enormity of his grief, which he expresses in his near-total loss of responsiveness to human warmth, but also because he compels us to ask the question: How can such a thing happen?—to Nazerman, to any of us? What causes a person to lose contact with himself so profoundly that he can no longer function with awareness of what is missing? How can one exist so utterly alone?

Because of the Holocaust, because he was forced to watch as his wife and children were shot to death by Nazi soldiers, because he was forced to live in the savagery of death camps, the entirety of the world of experience that had formerly defined Sol Nazerman's life was obliterated: its images, feelings, and the people who inhabited it, including himself—as an internal reality, not just as an external presence. As a consequence, Nazerman's psychological injury was reflected in and followed by a physiological loss of function. His memory, his ability to smile, his ability to

CHAPTER 7: LEGACIES: THE BRAIN, THE WILL, AND THE BODY

cry, or to feel physical pain were sheared from his functional control. There was no longer an external or internal reference to call on. His feelings of love, of grief, or of joy belonged to that other, former world of people and of himself in relation to them. Thus, he was left bereft: a stranger in a strange land, not only alien to others but to himself. He behaved as an automaton, his body following the demands of simple routines; but "he" was no longer connected to that body. Intrusions by people provoked his irritation, as one might swat at an annoying fly.

Nazerman's experience is a mirror image of that experienced by Oliver Sacks in the wake of the traumatic injury to his leg. Sacks found that he could not will his leg to move, much less to walk, even though surgery had repaired the torn muscles and nerves. The task was simple, yet far exceeded his capacities. Nor could Sol Nazerman will himself to participate in normal human interactions of friendship or pleasurable activities, both of which had been possible before his traumatic injury. Such demands called on vital connections between his thoughts and feelings, emotions and body, between his body and thoughts—connections that had been severed with the murder of his family and the destruction of his life.

The legacies of traumatic injury reflect the traumatic wounds that gave rise to them. The fragmentation of the structures of the self—which occurs during the traumatic process and culminates in the experience of utter loss, abandonment, and aloneness—is not easily repaired. Although some areas of "normal" function may return soon after safety is regained and basic life-sustaining functions of the body achieve stability, nevertheless, full reintegration of the self may take years or decades to accomplish, if at all.

The loss of wholeness and identity can be the most painful of all aspects of the aftermath of trauma. To become a stranger to oneself is confusing and frightening. One may retain an internal awareness that "something is missing," or, "I was not like this before." To find the missing pieces may require re-entry into the traumatic experience, through memory, which a person may or may not wish to undertake. Only each unique individual can assess the difficulties that may be involved in setting out on a search to find and reconnect the missing pieces of traumatic experience, both internal and external, since there is a danger that one can become overwhelmed anew in an encounter with one's own suffering. The presence of compassionate guides and helpers can offer a steadying force and provide a navigational compass to mark the way out of the void.

CHAPTER 8

Finding the Face of Compassion

"The best we can do is lean toward the light, toward the harmonious relationships that come from compassion with suffering, from understanding the other person."
—JOSEPH CAMPBELL

As Gretel Ehrlich struggled to maintain consciousness in the days and months after she was struck by lightning, her basic desire was simple: "I wanted to be held, to be pieced back together and fastened to the realm of the living by another human being."

She describes the moment when she first saw Blaine Braniff, her cardiologist, through the fog of her cardiac collapse and uncertain recovery: "When I looked up, my doctor was standing over me. He had unarmored eyes I could look into, and before I was able to speak, he made me smile." With each ensuing visit he "pulled me back into life…his curiosity and enthusiasm made me want to be alive.…"

"There is a chemistry," Ehrlich writes, "between the healer and the one being healed.…Perhaps the tenderness I felt toward him was also a tenderness I was able to feel toward myself."

The great gift of empathic care lies in the generous, forceful, tender, and lively presence of the healer, in whose face the wounded person may see a reflection of herself. Like other great physicians and healers, Blaine understood that Ehrlich and his other patients would tell him what he needed to know about their wounds; his job was to be fully present, to listen, and to respond with accuracy to what was being asked of him.

The quality of the interaction between Gretel Ehrlich and her doctor is an example of what any one of us might aspire to in efforts to help another person in the wake of traumatic collapse. Ehrlich experienced her relationship with Blaine as deeply collaborative. His eyes were "unarmored," she said; through them he allowed her access to him, and what she found was "curiosity" and "enthusiasm." It was as though she were being invited by this stranger, her doctor, to dance. Out of the loneliness of near-death, Ehrlich was invited to take the arm of someone who knew the steps of this unfamiliar dance, who could lead her to understand the new rhythms she must learn to follow, and who would allow her the grace and pleasure of becoming a full partner in helping her broken body into new patterns of life. At first she could only return the invitation with a smile or a word. Later she could stand and reach out her arm. Finally, she was able to move slowly across the terrain of her new surroundings, held safely in the frame provided by her partner—the doctor, the healer.

Guide, Witness, and Healer

No matter how much one might wish to take away the suffering of another, bearing witness to it, being present with one's whole attention and responding to what is needed with the tools and skills available is the best anyone can do. Sometimes there is only the ordinary with which to respond to tragedy and loss: a cup of coffee, faltering words, shared silence, or a gentle touch on the shoulder. And even the ordinary can seem so inadequate when the tragedy is very large.

This was my experience some years ago when I was called to assist two men, a father and son, who struggled to express their grief and to find meaning and comfort in the wake of their terrible loss.

CHAPTER 8: FINDING THE FACE OF COMPASSION

The son's wife had been murdered only a few days before in the parking lot of a suburban supermarket, a block away from the apartment where I met with the two men. She had been shot through the belly with a rifle, quickly killing her and her unborn nine-month-old child. The assailant was her first husband. He shot himself also and died nearby. He left a note and his diaries at the scene, which chronicled his previous months of secretly stalking his pregnant ex-wife, his obsession to keep her as his own, and his rage that culminated in her murder.

As I sat with the father, a career Marine officer in his late sixties, at a table in his son's small apartment kitchen, cradling cups of hot coffee in our hands, the son struggled to compose a eulogy for his wife, pacing from room to room. His grief, his pain, and his rage could not be contained or expressed in mere words.

There was nothing in the experience of the father or the son that could help them find meaning, understanding, or context in which to place the murder of this beloved young woman and her unborn child. As if in a daze, the father intoned: "It just doesn't fit," shaking his head slowly, as though from that small movement he could wrest some sense from this terrible loss. "It doesn't fit." These were the only words with which to express his sense of dislocation and disorientation. Nothing, not even combat as a Marine, had prepared him for this experience.

At moments like this there are no right words, no perfect gesture, no counsel to heal the injury of such loss. Being there, being present, bearing witness to the pain of these two men is all I had to offer.

The helplessness one feels in the face of such a tragedy can make a person want to turn away. It can cause a person to stay away altogether and not offer help or companionship, for fear it will not be enough, for fear it will be inadequate. To share in a moment of helplessness and defeat, dislocation and disorientation, can be frightening. Yet the connection one offers to those stunned by grief with a world outside of the tragedy can be lifesaving. One's simple presence may affirm the possibility of continuing life.

When I left the apartment, I walked to my car, distracted, at a loss to know what can be said that might have value in such a situation. Deep in thought, I was startled by a group of little boys, around the age of nine or so, swarming toward me with large, plastic guns pointed directly at my head and upper body. In mock attack they made explosive sounds with their mouths, as they ran toward me. I was struck dumb. What could I say to them that would make any sense in their world? They believed they were playing a game. They were only pretending to shoot me. But why would they want to shoot me in their game? The violence of their actions merged in my thoughts and feelings with the violence of the tragedy of the young woman's murder. My sense of utter helplessness to console or comfort the two men in their grief or to tell the little boys that violence is not a game cemented the certainty that this day would never leave my memory.

As witness to the suffering of others, the healer becomes a part of their suffering and is changed by it. There is no way to serve as a guide and remain outside of the traumatic experience. That doesn't mean that the helper must also become overwhelmed in order to assist the person who is overcome by traumatic loss or injury. On the contrary, it is essential that the helper try to keep at least one foot or thought or feeling outside of the traumatic experience, in order to provide an anchor in safe harbor as the storm sweeps through.

For those who set out to help others who have experienced profound trauma or who find themselves taking the part of healer quite by accident or circumstance, the work is both simple and extraordinarily difficult. The simple part is to communicate one's desire to know what pain or sorrow is afflicting the wounded person. "Tell me," one might say, "what is causing you such pain. Tell me what you need." The most difficult part is to listen, with all senses attuned, to the answers the wounded person needs to express, not the ones we might wish or expect to hear. Sometimes, when silence is the only answer available, the challenge is to understand

CHAPTER 8: FINDING THE FACE OF COMPASSION

that silence and create a relationship with it. It does no good and can even cause harm to try to alter the silence or the answers that are given to us.

In my many years of practice as a psychotherapist specializing in trauma, I learned from my clients, as Blaine had learned from his patients, the necessity of providing two key elements in our work together: safety and respectful collaboration. Without these we would find no trust with each other, and we would be defeated by the despair and fragmenting effects of trauma.

Despite good intentions, however, I found that I could not always guarantee the feeling of safety that I know is necessary for healing to proceed. External events that produce danger, such as earthquakes or violence or poverty or war, can interfere. And then there is the matter of poor judgment.

I recall the embarrassment and foolishness I felt, quite a few years ago, when I realized that the beautiful new office I had leased in a prestigious, historic, center-city building aroused panic and dread in many of my clients. What to me and many other office tenants of the building was an architectural delight created by the soaring, six-story atrium, instead created what looked to my clients like a cavernous, vertiginous, unwelcome hole in the building's center that was all-too-reflective of the hole in their own fragile cores. To top it off, only a thin railing separated the hallway to my office door from the wide gap of the atrium. It would not be hard to imagine one's unsteady, fragmented body falling headlong into the space below. The final insult to my clients was the elevator: an old-fashioned kind that consisted of a tiny, simple cage of glass walls providing an uncertain, bumpy ride.

Within a month of moving into the building I canceled my lease and found new quarters. Soon I moved into a solid building outside of the center of the city. Snugly placed in a friendly courtyard, it looked and felt like a home. It was firmly rooted in a diverse neighborhood of shops, houses, and lively pedestrians, and it put forward no obstacles to the already-hard work in which we were engaged. Quite the contrary: the new office and the building and neighborhood in which it was situated felt safe, welcoming, and calming.

Safety can be communicated in a building, in the setting of an office, and in the "unarmored" honesty of the healer. The question of safety takes on particular importance in trauma work because the nature of trauma itself includes danger. Remembering that the traumatic process often begins with a "surrender to inevitable danger," one can understand that the perception of danger—in a physical situation or communicated in the attitude or body language of another person—can trigger terrible traumatic memories. First and foremost, if one wishes to assist a person who has experienced any kind of trauma, the physical and practical safety of the wounded person must be addressed. Such safety issues may require finding shelter, food, and basic needs. In some situations it means finding a safe living situation away from violence and abuse. It always means getting out of harm's way, for both the helper and the wounded person.

In the widely differing kinds of offices or settings where I have provided counseling, in large cities and small towns, in fancy buildings and in storefront clinics, people entrusted me with their stories of sorrow, of loss, of terror, and of utter aloneness.

At certain times, when a story began to emerge in vivid starkness, as though it were occurring at that very moment in our presence, I would position our chairs so that we could face the story head-on, witnessing it together on an imaginary stage or screen in front of us. Seated so that our chairs were angled to be almost side-by-side, we watched as the words and silences emerged to make a picture. We listened and bore witness to the unfolding of a story that was too full of fear and pain and grief for one person to bear alone.

In the safe space of the consulting room, in the routine of our meetings, and in the story-telling itself, hope and determination to overcome terror and suffering were nourished. Together we would work to draw the ever-circling story of the experience of trauma safely into our hands, holding it tenderly as we would a frightened bird, and we would search to find a place for it finally to come to rest in the history of events of the past. Together we would allow the timid possibility of a future to emerge.

The physician, counselor, close friend, or relative, even a stranger may find him- or herself assigned the role of the leader of a team assisting the trauma survivor. Without understanding the meaning, the force, and the impact of this responsibility, he or she may inadvertently undermine the confidence of the wounded person, invalidate his strengths, and abandon him to fear and suffering. This was the case with Oliver Sacks' experience in the London hospital after his fall and injury on the mountain in Norway. The surgeon and the resident physician in charge of his care would only look at the ligaments and tissues, sutures and dressings. They refused to look at their patient's psychological experience as it related to his neurological injuries and help him to interpret and understand his experience. Sacks' perceptions were invalidated and his desire to collaborate with his doctors was denied. This set the tone for the kind of care provided by the entire team entrusted with his recovery at the hospital. Sacks was essentially abandoned.

Failures of Compassion

Although I believe that reaching out to provide connection, protection, and strength are spontaneous responses intrinsic to life, it is clear that failures of compassion can and do occur frequently. The consequences of such failures can lead to further injury or death. For this reason it's important to explore some of the attitudes, feeling states, and even misunderstandings that can limit or thwart the basic ability to give compassion and help to a traumatized person.

Fear and Fatigue

It may seem strange to imagine that those entrusted with the care of others might be frightened: frightened of pain, frightened of witnessing wounds, frightened of feelings—their own or others'. For instance, it is probably not uncommon that physicians who are trained to "cut and sew" may not have been trained to administer empathy. In fact, such medical specializations often encourage practitioners to put aside personal feeling and to provide dispassionate service. Unfortunately, a common defense against a feeling of unfamiliarity or unpreparedness to deal with the care of a traumatized person may be to assign inaccurate "causes" for the problems being expressed. Thus, like Oliver Sacks, a patient might be told, incorrectly, "it's all in your head; you're making this up; your experience (or lack of experience) of your body is not believable."

Since traumatic experience engendered by emotional abuse or distress often has a strong somatic or bodily component, the physical symptoms that express the experience of abuse may be neglected as though they are "not real," leading to serious health consequences.

Holistic medicine, on the other hand, attempts to understand and respond to the complex interactions and connections between all systems of the individual person, including the psychological, the physical, the cognitive, and the spiritual. Without such comprehensive training and outlook, a practitioner may not be able to respond to certain aspects of illness, leading to a failure of compassionate connection that is so important to any healing relationship.

Another impediment to compassionate response may occur when too much pain or too much sorrow and injury make constant demands on one's resources and strengths, rendering a person, a family, or even a nation overwhelmed and exhausted. "Compassion fatigue" is one name that has been given to this experience of a surfeit of woundedness through empathic connection with others.

CHAPTER 8: FINDING THE FACE OF COMPASSION

Physicians, counselors, disaster workers, nurses, or family and community caregivers can experience compassion fatigue. It can render a person incapable of asserting the most basic empathic responses, even to a friend or loved one. Otherwise caring people can feel helpless to provide meaningful responses to others in obvious need and experience guilt and shame as a result. There is no easy remedy for this problem. Sometimes there is no letup from demands on one's compassion, as in times of national tragedy, natural disaster, or family illness and loss. Yet any condition of fatigue can be helped by rest. It becomes essential to take time away from responsibilities of caregiving in order to restore and nourish one's own integrity and strengths. If compassion fatigue, like any other kind of fatigue, is ignored for too long, the consequences can be unhealthy and even dangerous.

Additionally, if the healer or guide has been wounded himself, often it is necessary to overcome terrible dread to assist another who is suffering. There is always the latent fear that one can be overwhelmed once again, pulled into the vortex of the traumatic process. Just the fear of such a recurrence may be enough to cause a person to freeze or turn away from offering help. Wounded healers may provide great compassionate care to others who, like them, have been traumatized. However, they must take great care to respect their own vulnerabilities and not ignore the particular difficulties they face in once again confronting traumatic experience.

Attitudes toward Death

The story of Beck Weathers' miraculous survival on Mount Everest in 1996 is not complete without a discussion of the failure of compassion of other climbers, which nearly defeated Weathers' solitary efforts to survive. One has to wonder, what caused the other climbers to abandon Weathers where he lay on the side of the mountain? What allowed them to walk away from Yasuko Namba, the Japanese woman climber who lay next to Weathers, allowing her to die? And what caused them to abandon Weathers a second time after he had finally reached the safety of camp?

Were the other climbers afraid of death itself? These people who lived with the possibility of death at every step of their climb up Everest may have felt unequal to the task of just being in the presence of death, feeling their own helplessness, and believing there was nothing they could do but to witness death's steady progress. If they were to fully recognize the reality of death, could they continue their climb?

Remembering how Weathers appeared as he staggered into the High Camp, Todd Burleson said: "I couldn't believe what I saw. This man had no face. It was completely black, solid black, like he had a crust over him. His jacket was unzipped down to his waist, full of snow. His right arm was bare and frozen over his head. We could not lower it. His skin looked like marble. White stone. No blood in it."

Weathers was a dead man, though still walking. Fearful of this apparition and following medical advice from base camp that asserted Weathers was beyond help, the other climbers put Weathers in a tent, without food or friends or comfort, and for a second time left him for dead.

A new storm engulfed the camp during the night and filled Weathers' tent with snow. In the morning, hearing the voices of the last climbers who were hurriedly breaking camp to descend the mountain, he roused himself to consciousness for a moment and called out: "Hello, anybody out there?" Then, to an astonished fellow climber, who peered into the tent at "the dead man," Weathers said: "What the hell does a person have to do around here to get a little service!"

The familiar joking tone of voice that they recognized as their indomitable climbing companion stirred the others to break away from their belief that Weathers was already doomed to death, and they begin to assist him to live.

Beck Weathers' wife, Peach, addresses the issue of the other climbers' actions this way:

CHAPTER 8: FINDING THE FACE OF COMPASSION

— *I can sort of understand why no one was able or willing to risk their lives to rescue Beck or Yasuko. I even sort of understand the medical edict from Base Camp that Beck should be left to die at High Camp. What I don't understand is why they left him alone in that tent overnight....I've thought this over again and again. Where was their basic human compassion? Being in the tent with Beck certainly would not have endangered anyone. If they figured he was going to die, then being there to hear his final words, and perhaps pass them on to those he left behind, would have been a tremendous comfort to us.*

Exploring these same questions regarding the failure of compassion that occurs all too frequently in the current world of commercial, competitive mountaineering, Joe Simpson writes:

— *Does all this [commercialization of climbing Everest] necessarily mean we are bound in the end to behave inhumanely? I cannot push from my mind those two incidents when climbers abandoned their fellow climbers to die alone and made no effort to give aid or comfort, however futile it may have seemed....No summit can ever be worth so much. No man should be able to witness such harrowing events and not be moved to help. Or am I biased, knowing how it feels to be left for dead?*

At any stage of life and health, a person must be accorded respect, and the value of his life must be affirmed. But if a person, even a society, is afraid of death and cannot tolerate being in the presence of death or of a dying person, then the individual and the community are bound to act inhumanely.

Bernard Lown, a noted cardiologist and Nobel Peace Laureate, suggests that the same principles of care apply to the frail elderly and to those who are facing the end of their lives, as to a person in the prime of life. He writes that "Death should not deplete in one's last days the dignified sense of self that took a lifetime to cultivate." Death need not be a fearful spectre, Lown asserts, if one is assured that he or she will not be abandoned and that those providing companionship and care will do all they can to mitigate pain.

In many ways the needs of the dying person differ only a little from the needs of a woman giving birth. If both death and birth are understood as efforts to create and give expression to a new life, then the difficulties encountered in each can be managed. Both processes entail withdrawal into a private place to accomplish the task at hand, and both benefit from the assistance of a witness (also known as a doula, a guide, a shaman, an anamcara) to steady the way through to the other side of the experience. The helper may be called on to provide physical assistance or simply to be present, and by her very presence she provides assurance that the person in her care will not be abandoned.

The Core of Strength

The compassionate counselor, physician, friend, or helper is a guide who leads the woman giving birth, the wounded victim of disaster, the injured or the dying person to connection with his or her own deepest strengths. In order to do this, the healer must also be firmly connected with his own strengths. Through the interconnection of the core strengths of both healer and wounded comes the ability to create a vision of new life. Jerome Groopman explains what he understands as the essential aspects of his role as a physician and guide in this way:

— *You show...that there is a strategy in place...and you search for the core of their strength. You need to find this, to nurture it, because it will be sorely tested.... You need to understand this inner strength, where it comes from, how deep and resilient it is. Once you find it and comprehend it, you try to take it in your hand and fuse it with your own, because together this creates the unified force required to sustain the patient.*

CHAPTER 8: FINDING THE FACE OF COMPASSION

The body seeks what it needs to regain its equilibrium and strength of function. However, if there has been interference, from illness or injury or damage to one's confidence and connection with one's body, the physician, care provider, or friend may often be called on to help re-invigorate the urge toward integrative action, which lies dormant within.

The work of A. Jean Ayers, Ph.D., O.T.R., suggests that human beings have an innate drive to become integrated, that is to experience an inner unity based on neurological coordination and modulation of sensory input. Ayers, born in 1920, was an occupational therapist who developed in the 1970s the theory and practice of Sensory Integration to assist children exhibiting symptoms of neurological injury resulting in learning and behavioral difficulties. Her research and the therapeutic tools based on her theory of Sensory Integration continue to assist people of all ages to build on the integrated strengths of the basic sensory systems. At the heart of her work is the understanding that an injured, fragmented person has the primary need to achieve soothing and calming through activities that work on a sub-cortical level in the central nervous system to achieve this effect. Such integrating activities lead to a sense of safety and provide the foundation on which to build new strength, confidence, and skills.

For instance, mothers have long known that the gentle, rhythmic movement of a rocking chair provides a wonderful activity of calming and soothing for a fretful baby, as well as for themselves. Recently, I met a young man severely afflicted with hallucinations and chronic agitation who explained that his rocking chair provides him a place of refuge and great comfort. It's no accident that children (and adults, too) love the motion of swings. The rhythmic, swaying motions found in dancing, ironing clothes, bowling, and washing a car may serve to forestall panic and terror. Gardening offers the experience of bowing, dipping, and lifting one's head and upper body with a bonus of the tactile pleasure and stimulation of hands in the earth.

All of these movements achieve their integrative benefits by their stimulation of the tactile, proprioceptive, and vestibular systems and the consequent effects on the central nervous system. But it isn't necessary to know how these activities work in order for them to be useful in providing comfort and modulation of the extreme states caused by traumatic experience. More important is the helper's validation of each individual's unique personal understanding of preferred activities. What "works" for one person may cause distress for another.

Most people know intuitively what are uniquely their own choices of preferred, integrative activities; however, they seldom are called on to name them or consider the reasons for their usefulness. When psychological and/or physiological stress or injury challenge the body's ability to function in an integrated, coordinated manner, taking an inventory of these spontaneous actions and bringing them into service can lead to important achievements in the ability to regain "normal" functioning.

In an amusing anecdote, Oliver Sacks describes his first interview with his lively and somewhat unconventional orthopedist. Sacks was depressed at his lack of progress in reintegrating the perception of his injured leg and his ability to use it normally. In response to the orthopedist's inquiry as to what activities he enjoyed, Sacks responded that he liked to swim. The orthopedist right then conspired by telephone with a lifeguard colleague at a nearby pool to trick Sacks into spontaneous re-integrative movement.

When Sacks arrived at the pool a short time later, the lifeguard chatted with him and then gave Sacks a surprise nudge into the water, forcing him to overcome his fear that his leg would not work properly and to swim spontaneously. It was this event that resulted in the final re-integration of his damaged leg into his body's memory of moving, walking, and of being whole. What he had not been able to accomplish with imagination, with memory, or with reason, Sacks was finally able to achieve in the spontaneous movements and rhythms of swimming—with the help of a crafty doctor and lifeguard.

Many people, like Gretel Ehrlich, identify walking as an important and pleasurable integrative and restorative activity. When Ehrlich was still

CHAPTER 8: FINDING THE FACE OF COMPASSION

too ill even to stride across her small room, much less to hike her favorite mountain trails, she spent hours in reveries of walking, accompanied by recordings of music that set the rhythm. Some believe that walking is a core strength in and of itself because of our nomadic origins—that the rhythm of walking is embedded in our genetic memory—that it is integrative not only for the body, but also for one's sense of continuity of self within the history of the human family. I must confess that I, too, experience an imperative to walk, especially when complex or distressing experiences weigh on my thoughts and agitate my body. The rhythm of walking supercedes restless thought and allows for new connections between mind and body and emotions, opening a space for creative solutions. *Solvitur ambulando*: "it is solved in walking."

Just as the compassionate healer may ask: "What pain is causing you to suffer so?" the healer might also ask, "What do you enjoy?…What gives you delight?" These are compassionate questions, born of a genuine interest in the other person. Such questions don't deny the pain of suffering; their intention is to provide an opportunity to identify and to validate a person's basic strengths that will enable him or her to endure. In the answers to these simple questions a person may find the pathways that lead from despair and fragmentation to hopefulness and integration.

And there are times when no words and no questions are necessary, only the simple action of providing what is clearly needed. At such times there is a deep interconnection of energies of life that are exchanged in a moment of complete trust.

Such a moment was described by Antoine de Saint-Exupéry in the short passage that follows, found in his book *Wind, Sand and Stars*.

The Face of All Mankind

Lost in the Libyan desert, having survived the crash landing of their plane, Antoine de Saint-Exupéry and his co-pilot Prevot had wandered for days, walking over one hundred twenty miles. Finally, Saint-Exupéry realized that they had come to the end of their abilities to maintain their own lives. Without food or water their bodies were rapidly turning to dust in the desert. Without sorrow or hope they trudged on.

At this moment of utter loss and loneliness, suddenly, incredibly, Saint-Exupéry saw in the sand in front of him footprints. This time he was sure they were not their own footsteps circling back on themselves. Remembering what happened next, he writes:

— *We had wandered from the trail of the human species; we had cast ourselves forth from the tribe; we had found ourselves alone on earth and forgotten by the universal migration; and here, imprinted in the sand, were the divine and naked feet of man!...*

The miracle had come to pass. He [the Bedouin] was walking towards us over the sand like a god over the waves....

The Arab looked at us without a word. He placed his hands upon our shoulders and we obeyed him: we stretched out upon the sand. Race, language, religion were forgotten. There was only this humble nomad with the hands of an archangel on our shoulders.

Face to the sand, we waited. And when the water came, we drank like calves with our faces in the basin....

You, Bedouin of Libya who saved our lives, though you will dwell for ever in my memory yet I shall never be able to recapture your features. You are Humanity and your face comes into my mind simply as a man incarnate. You, our beloved fellow man, did not know who we might be, and yet you recognized us without fail. And I, in my turn, shall recognize you in the faces of all mankind. You came towards me in an aureole of charity and magnanimity bearing the gift of water. All my friends and all my enemies marched towards me in your person. It did not seem to me that you were rescuing me: rather it did seem that you were forgiving me. And I felt I had no enemy left in all the world.

CHAPTER 9

Pieces Come Together

"Nature is not only all that is visible to the eye—it also includes the inner pictures of the soul."
—EDVARD MUNCH

The presence of a compassionate witness or healer can bring light and touch, voice and hope into the darkness and utter aloneness of traumatic injury and its aftermath. The face of compassion may be that of a stranger who provides a cup of water or a doctor who listens to the sorrow of wounds and dresses them with care or a friend who extends a gentle hand on the shoulder. Each becomes a companion for life, an anchor to human connection that one can hold onto when sudden storms return. Each provides the connecting link with one's deepest humanity, reflecting one's strengths and vulnerabilities, mercy and determination, one's fragility and desire.

The presence of compassion may also be experienced in the song of a bird, in the soothing breath of wind on one's face, in the solid strength of the flank of a mountain, or the constancy of the river's flow. These are companions also, reflecting a sense of order and wholeness, of endurance and transformation. They are a comfort when one's own small part of life seems fractured and incoherent and are a reminder of a larger, intricately woven structure of life to which we belong.

In the presence of compassion, one can find the courage to gather together the pieces of a broken life and allow new meaning and direction to emerge.

The Beauty of a Rock

One afternoon a few years ago, sitting on the steps at my sister's home, I found myself telling one of her friends, a stranger to me, about my mother's life of pain and fear and about a rock I had recently found that had taken on special meaning for me. As I embarked on this conversation, I had no conscious idea of how the two stories—of my mother's life and of my relationship with the rock—fit together. I didn't know where these thoughts were leading me; they seemed to have a life of their own. The man who sat beside me listening was a gentle witness. By the ease of his presence he encouraged me to follow the separate strands of my narrative to the point of their connection, and in doing so I found new insight. In this simple, undramatic moment I found resolution to what had been a great burden of traumatic wounding for over fifty years. The story I told him was this:

Almost every day, over the course of several years, my dog Babe and I visited a local park where we trained on practice trails for Search and Rescue. As a reward for our hard work, we then took long walks beyond the park boundaries into rolling hills and broad meadows, enjoying the quiet and beauty. I found that the natural rhythm of walking allowed my thoughts and emotions to rest. Not infrequently I would emerge from one of our long walks with new understandings of problems that had been nagging at me when I first set out.

One day, while following a familiar jeep trail, I noticed a pile of large stones that gleamed in the sunlight. One rock in particular caught my attention. It was a boulder, really, maybe three feet high and two-and-a-half feet wide. It was perched on top of a gigantic gopher warren and was

CHAPTER 9: PIECES COME TOGETHER

surrounded by other huge rocks. This piece of serpentine had surfaces of shining silver-green with deep bands of blue and jade-green running through it.

I began to visit the rock each time Babe and I went to the fields for a walk. It seemed to call me into connection. I would stop and run my hand across its upper face that had been smoothed by wind and weather. Leaning against its side, listening to meadowlarks and watching the circling flight of hawks, it seemed to speak to me.

For a long time I wanted to own this rock, to tame it. I imagined bringing in a bulldozer to dig it out of its place and load it on a truck. I wanted to take it to my home to set out in my fields. But its surface layers were brittle, and I realized that its beautiful face would chip and crumble if it was disturbed. It was only after many visits that I was able to accept that this rock had to stay where I found it. It had its own place and reason for being where it was.

Gradually, I became aware that my urge to move the rock from its place, to change it, even at the risk of damaging its integrity, resembled my long-held wish to change my mother: to move her away from the terrors and pain of trauma and to bring her closer to me. I wished for a different kind of relationship with my mother, one not dominated by traumatic experience but one in which comfort, empathy, and joy could find expression. But these tender feelings had been banished, along with the dread and terror that were legacies of her vulnerability. It had always been a source of grief and loneliness to me that my mother and I were bound together mainly by unspoken fears, mistrust, and shame: the aftereffects of trauma, her own and those she passed on to me.

"I am a rock, I don't have feelings," my mother would often say. And I would argue then, as I do now, that rocks and trees and rivers and even a blade of grass indeed have feelings, and so did she. For my mother, however, the word "feelings" meant only the pain and terror she associated with her experiences of trauma. For this reason she was desperate to be free from feeling, to deny feelings altogether. They could only lead to disappointment and profound grief.

My mother's death, over a decade ago, finally fulfilled her yearning to be free from the emotional and physical pain that haunted her most of her life. For me also, her death released at last the bonds of trauma, bonds that had held us in defensive positions: both of us on guard, frightened of becoming overwhelmed by the terror and dread that always lingered in the air but could not be spoken of.

Now, in this dusty field, I found that the fears and anguish of my mother's life, which I had carried also, were transformed and given expression in the iridescent beauty of the serpentine stone. Her hidden strength was now visible to me in the form of this rock, and I was able to stand next to her in safety. The beautiful serpentine boulder had a different message for me. "We are our separate selves, changed and changing," the rock said. "You can stand and rest beside me now, and I won't bring you any harm."

The fragments of this story swirled in my thoughts in unconnected pieces for some time. It wasn't until I spoke them aloud, until they were heard and validated and witnessed by the silent acceptance and gentle smile of the stranger, that I was able to understand my own experience with the rock that had spoken to me. The pieces of the story came together in a meaningful form as I spoke them aloud: thoughts, feelings, spiritual awareness, and physical experience of the world united into one deeply personal understanding. The rock, my mother, and I had been transformed, and I found joy in our being together. What relief to have these pieces finally make a whole picture. I felt a sense of completion. At last I felt safe.

This is often how it is—that traumatic experience and its legacies are resolved in the slow wearing away of time: the rough edges and spurs of suffering are worn smooth with the relentless press of wind and rain, of

CHAPTER 9: PIECES COME TOGETHER

sun, and the mere weight of being. What is revealed is the inner beauty that has always been there but has been hidden, seen only in brief glimpses of insight and ephemeral epiphanies along the way.

Something Is Terribly Wrong

Having finally come to a resolution of my personal experience of family trauma, I was quite ready to enjoy the calm that ensued. I welcomed the prospect of no more turbulence and no more underlying sadness. Ironically, however, the resolution of past pain seemed to have created an opportunity to recognize present difficulties. Despite the well-being that permeated my everyday life, an awareness emerged—one that had been waiting just out of sight to make itself known—that something was terribly wrong.

As I began to listen and look and open my senses with greater attention, I found that within my own experience and all around me warning bells were sounding more loudly each day, reaching a din that could not be ignored. Small incidents and large portrayed a picture of traumatic experience in progress, and I was part of it. I realized that a new sense of deep grief and of fear-bordering-on-terror were never far from my consciousness. Information and intuition came together to affirm that something was and is deeply amiss in the relationship between our human activities and the health of our physical environment.

Stories of everyday life report with increasing frequency the relentless destruction of open spaces and habitat for diverse species of animals and plants, on land and in the water. Newspapers tell of forests, even entire mountains, cut down to meet human demand. Scientific articles document the phenomenon and consequences of global warming. The mounting death toll of entire species of plants, trees, and animals are recorded daily in public media, with the unmistakable underlying message that the demise of the human species cannot be far behind.

Also documented is a new kind of human violence, both interpersonal and suicidal, taking place on a global scale. The warning is clear: it is a dangerous luxury, no longer affordable, to hold onto the belief that the violence and losses occurring in the natural environment are unrelated to the violence and losses occurring in the human community. What is less clear is what can be done to stop the common downward spiral of environmental and human well-being.

To respond to the accretion of evidence of our collective peril and to my own deep worry and grief for what we have lost and what we are losing, I have felt drawn to make a commitment to a new search. This new search requires an exploration of the intersection between human traumatic experience and trauma occurring in the environment. What has been lost are the essential connections that have shaped and held together a unified co-existence between human life and the rest of the natural world, animate and inanimate. Human life and non-human life have become separated and lost from one another: both are profoundly wounded.

Remember for a moment the colors and images used earlier (in Chapter 3) to describe the course of the traumatic process. As one's vital connections with family, loved ones, social networks, place of belonging, and meaning are severed, one is left utterly alone, a fading light in a world turned dark all around. This image describes also our collective loss of connection with what is beloved, what nourishes and gives us life, what provides us with structure and meaning—with our natural environment. And does the world of nature mourn the loss of connection with us, also? I imagine so, but we have forgotten how to listen. Collectively, our memory has faded—we have forgotten family and where to find our home. We are walking down a dark path; the night is growing colder.

The success of the search to restore connection—to bring wholeness and integrity to our lives, natural and human—depends on the application of diverse skills and abilities of many: human and non-human alike. All senses are required. The search is urgent.

CHAPTER 9: PIECES COME TOGETHER

Everyday Signs and Symptoms

It is almost impossible to hold in one's thoughts the enormous, cataclysmic projections and predictions about our collective human and environmental fate that one now hears and experiences daily. The threats of global warming, of ice caps melting and seas rising, of famine and pandemics, of nuclear annihilation and global terrorism, seem too vast, too much like science fiction to grasp. One recoils at the task of comprehending such facts. Even small, day-to-day events and personal experiences, however, remind one of the losses taking place in our environment—and can accumulate and prove to be overwhelming.

The following story, told to me by a friend a few years ago, is an example of how personal experience reflects and reminds us of our communal experience. It is emblematic of our collective woundedness and grief in relation to our environmental degradation and loss.

Driving her eight-year-old son home from school one afternoon, Louise stopped her car at a familiar intersection where the town's boundary line and rolling countryside meet at the foot of a hill. This little hill is the smallest and the gentlest of the "Seven Sisters," a chain of morros that have volcanic origins and serve as signature landmarks of our rural community. As the boy let his gaze rise to the familiar contours of the hill, he let out a cry and began to weep with grief. While he had been at school, bulldozers had carved away a large section of the side of the hill to prepare for a housing development. The sight of the deep gash, the wound in the torso of the hill, caused the boy real pain. He felt the cut in the earth as though he or someone he loved had been injured. This smallest of the Seven Sisters was wounded. Her integrity, the wholeness of the hill as he had come to know it and appreciate it each day as he went to and from school, was forever lost. My friend could find no words with which to console her son.

Children understand and experience directly a kinship with the natural world they inhabit. One has only to watch children at play to observe their intense curiosity in all that creeps and crawls and flies and flutters and oozes and burrows and sparkles and whistles and hisses and splashes and erupts. Children have long conversations with the moon, with ants, with trees, with stones, and myriad other visible and invisible aspects of the natural world. They receive comfort and an assurance of belonging in their interactions with their natural environment.

From worried adults, however, children are now learning to fear exposure to the sun, to fear drinking water from a stream, to regard the soil as dirty and toxic. These basic aspects of nature, which once were understood as being generative and sustaining, are now perceived as harmful. And there is cause for the worried alarms of adults. There is evidence that our relationship with the natural world, of which we are an integral part, is going terribly wrong: we are harming each other reciprocally and do not know how to stop.

Everywhere one looks, barren wastelands are replacing once rich and thriving communities of diverse species. Even a lush green suburban lawn becomes a wasteland when every creature living within the fabric of its structure is considered an enemy and is poisoned. The open plains of the eastern slopes of the Rocky Mountains—once a landscape that provided soothing silence, broken in the evening only by the sound of raptors calling as they scanned the fields for sustenance and in the morning by the songs of meadowlarks—have been replaced by houses, shopping malls, roads, and the roar of bulldozers, trucks, and automobiles. A brown haze of polluted air obscures a once-clear view of distant mountain peaks, a visual connection that in the past had provided rest and inspiration. Stories of such disrupted connections between human life and nature abound.

Contracts Are Broken

For over a quarter of a century the pioneering cardiologist and Nobel Peace Laureate Bernard Lown has been raising concerns that technology

CHAPTER 9: PIECES COME TOGETHER

and science threaten to overshadow an empathic understanding of human interrelatedness with all life. Not only have industrialized communities lost a basic connection with the environment on which their lives depend, Lown contends, but also the implicit contract between the healer and wounded individuals has been broken. "In my view," Lown writes, "medicine has lost its way, if not its soul. An unwritten covenant between doctor and patient, hallowed over several millennia, is being broken." The "medical-industrial complex," as Lown describes it, has replaced the concerned connection between healer and the distressed soul. The rules of business, technology, and science dictate the terms of the relationship between patient and healer, replacing the compassionate care that is called for.

In the rules of business, technology, and science that govern modern medicine, there is little room for affirming the essential connection between human and ecological health. A few years ago, when the journal *Science* reported that people recover more quickly in rooms with a window facing a tree, it was considered scientific news. "These patients," the study stated, "required a lesser dose of narcotics, healed faster, and were discharged from the hospital earlier than those randomly assigned to a room facing a desolate parking lot." How is it that we have forgotten what is most basic to our well-being? How have we come to forget that to confine an injured, frightened, or dying person to a sterile, sensory-deprived environment, only serves to compound the loss of connection that the individual already feels: that our health depends on our connection with the trees, with all of nature?

The broken contract between healer and patient referred to by Lown is only one of the visible signs of a more wide-reaching breach of relationships taking place on a global scale. Vast human populations now treat the natural environment as though we have no real relation to it. We bomb it, we carve it up, we detonate great shattering blasts at the bottom of the oceans, we stockpile toxic wastes under its sands, we dry up fresh water lakes, and we burn holes in our protective atmosphere. We do all this as though it, our natural environment, has nothing at all to do with us, as though our lives do not depend on the consequences of these actions.

Terry Tempest Williams, for many years the Naturalist-in-Residence at the Utah Museum of Natural History, provides compelling, personal evidence that abuse of our relationship with the land and our natural environment can and does result in loss of personal health and deep grief. After the death of her mother from breast cancer, Williams discovered that she belongs to a large community of people, including most of the women in her immediate and extended family, who have suffered the consequences of radioactive fallout from early nuclear testing in the Nevada desert. At the age of thirty-four, Williams became the matriarch of her family. All of her female elders had died of cancer.

It was only by accident that Williams learned that she, too, had been exposed to a nuclear bomb blast in the Nevada desert. One evening, not long after her mother's death, Williams happened to mention to her father a recurring image she had experienced since childhood that she could not erase from her mind's eye. It haunted and disturbed her. It was an image that had no reference in her memory, no validation in her reality. (We have learned that such images often carry the memories of trauma.) She explained to her father that often when she drove into the desert at night, a "flash of light" would fill her vision.

As she described this to her father, she assumed that she had fabricated the experience in her imagination. Her father startled her, however, with the information that she had, in fact, seen such a flash of light when she was a little girl, sitting on her mother's lap in the family car as they drove across Nevada in September of 1957. Her vision was a memory of a real event. Soon after the flash, her father said, they felt a concussion that rocked the car; they watched as a mushroom cloud rose from the desert floor; then ash rained down on the car. They had witnessed and experienced directly the explosion of a nuclear bomb.

CHAPTER 9: PIECES COME TOGETHER

The information that Williams learned from her father encouraged and strengthened her resolve to break the silence about the effects of the desert nuclear testing of the past and its legacy in the present. In the company of other women in 1988 Williams crossed the gates of the Nevada Test Site to stand on the wounded land: to bear witness in the desert to the interconnection between her own health, the lives of the women in her family, and that of the land at the heart of the country.

Williams explains: "A contract had been made and broken between human beings and the land. A new contract was being drawn by the women, who understood the fate of the earth as their own.... The time had come to protest with the heart, that to deny one's genealogy with the earth was to commit treason against one's soul."

Apocalyptic Visions

To remedy the grief experienced in relation to losses that are accumulating at a terrible speed, some people retreat rather than speak out. They are unable to take action and to reach out to others, as Bernard Lown and Terry Tempest Williams were able to do. Some stop looking beyond their own footsteps. Like emergency workers, they focus only on their own small part in the overall crisis in order to tolerate the terror and grief before them. Other people stop taking in further information: they stop reading papers or watching TV in order to avoid the daily accounts of human and environmental losses. Many people are fearful of succumbing to life-threatening despair, and they invent myriad ways to keep "busy," including the use of drugs that speed the metabolism or numb the senses.

Even more striking, however, is the silence. It has the weight and feel of the determined silence of people who have been terribly wounded: who do not dare speak for fear of being overcome by their own feelings, who fear they will injure others by speaking, or who believe it will only make matters worse if they reveal their dread and pain.

The current denial of the essential interconnection of all things is not a given of human nature. It represents a certain kind of human response that is born of fear, of dread, and of injury. By resemblance, such a response suggests to me that it is a legacy of traumatic wounding. Just as my mother's legacy of traumatic experience—her pain, her terror, and her dread expectation of the return of trauma—permeated the life of her family, with no storyline attached with which to understand it, so there is a legacy of trauma with which we now live. With determination and persistence it is possible to breach the barriers of silence and to name the injuries that afflict us. Only by doing so can we hope to find a way out of the grip of traumatic suffering. Failure to acknowledge our legacy of trauma leads us into extreme responses from which it becomes increasingly difficult to recover.

We know from studies of human traumatic injury that an accumulation of pain, of fear, and of hate can lead to a collapse of the structure of the individual self, just as surely as a building can be brought down by a bomb. Such a collapse is experienced as an internal wasteland in which life-sustaining connections are lost and the individual is cut off from himself and others and is utterly alone.

When the internal experience of a wasteland—the collapse of personal structures of identity, meaning, and autonomy—is mirrored by an external wasteland of social imbalance, environmental degradation and exploitation, and cataclysmic threats of global extinction, then individuals and societies may turn to apocalyptic visions for comfort and release. Suicidal thoughts, images, and actions may seem to the wounded person or community the only hope for a way out of the wasteland of despair.

Reflecting on his own experience and observations as a political prisoner in the Soviet Union during the 1980s, Natan Sharansky has said: "If life today seems meaningless, man inevitably makes himself see the end of it on a near horizon." Such a drive to end the despair of a life without

CHAPTER 9: PIECES COME TOGETHER

meaning can be understood as an expression of a traumatic process that can lead to self-inflicted death.

At this time in human history, such apocalyptic visions are expressed collectively as well as individually around the globe: from Japan to Indonesia to Saudi Arabia to Western Europe to the United States. A desire for new life, free from what appears to some to be inevitable danger and suffering, is given form in apocalyptic visions, images, and beliefs.

Robert Jay Lifton has written about this suicidal drive to put an end to the wasteland that has become a part of our present collective experience. In his analysis of the rise to power of Shōkō Asahara, the leader of the cult Aum Shinrikyō in Japan, Lifton explains:

— *There is a global sub-culture of apocalyptic violence—of violence conceived in sweeping terms as a purification and renewal of humankind through the total or near-total destruction of the planet.*

Increasingly widespread among ordinary people is the feeling of things going so wrong that only extreme measures can restore virtue and righteousness to society. When the world comes to be experienced as both hateful and dead or dying, a visionary guru can seize on such feelings while promising to replace them with equally absolute love and life-power.

While Shōkō Asahara annunciates an apocalyptic vision of redemptive violence in Japan, a world away Osama bin Laden, and those who follow in his footsteps, offer a vision of transcendence and transformation through self-destruction and mass violence. "Death is better than life in humiliation!" bin Laden has said. The apocalyptic visionaries hold out the hope of escape from the numbing decay of a world in which meaningful involvement and contribution seem impossible, where truth has become an expendable commodity, and purposeful endeavor seems destined to lead to further downward-spiraling of social balance and ecological health. Young men and women in many cultures, including our own, are vulnerable to promises of a better world beyond this life.

A parent in Saudi Arabia watches helplessly as his daughter is drawn in equal measure to Britney Spears and Osama bin Laden. The father understands his daughter's attraction to the former, but her dedication to the latter fills him with dread. "We are afraid of our children," the father explains. In another time, one might have been more likely to hear a father say: We are afraid *for* our children.

In Vermont in recent years a series of cold-blooded murders perpetrated by very young men has shaken the calm and confidence of a state that once represented an American ideal of social and moral order. In an essay on the Vermont murders that appeared in 2002 in *The Atlantic Monthly*, Ron Powers concludes:

— *To most people, the notion that an apocalyptic nihilism is taking root in this nation's children will seem alarmist.... We must ask ourselves today: "Why are so many children plotting to blow up their worlds and themselves?" For each act of gratuitous violence that is actually carried out, how many unconsummated dark fantasies are transmuted into depression, resignation, or a benumbed withdrawal from participation in civic society?*

Like Robert Jay Lifton, Powers asserts that "what we are witnessing is clearly something new." And Lifton echoes: "Outbreaks anywhere reverberate everywhere."

Young people carry not only the hope for their society but also the memories and consequences of its woundedness. At the heart of this new kind of apocalyptic violence, both homicidal and suicidal, is an effort to end traumatic suffering, a suffering that originates not with the young people who commit the acts of terror and brutality but suffering that

CHAPTER 9: PIECES COME TOGETHER

arises from pain, despair, and helplessness that has been transmitted to them by the larger communities, societies, and by the physical environment in which they live.

The boys of Vermont see themselves as heroes of a wasteland—a wasteland they did not create but that has been given to them. To fulfill the role of hero, they have learned to numb themselves to pain. Like Sol Nazerman, in the final scene of the movie *The Pawnbroker*, in which he purposely inflicts terrible pain on himself in a desperate attempt to rid himself of suffering, the boys attempt to construct an internal world beyond pain, beyond terror, in order to become masters of suffering. Their self-destruction is lived out in a form of psychogenic death. They have surrendered to the inevitable danger of a life without meaning, have embraced it, and cannot let go until something or someone comes along to break their desperate grip.

For the young followers of Asahara and bin Laden, who embrace violence and the possibility of self-destruction with a passion similar to the Vermont youth, a larger vision of transformation and transcendence fills their fantasies. Instead of numbness, they look forward to participating in an ecstatic destruction of the damaged and broken world giving them pain, with the hope and promise that a new and meaningful life will take its place. They believe they will find a place of honor in the new world that awaits them after their self-destruction.

The Cultural Imperative for Witnessing

As the warning signals and alarms grow louder and more urgent, a tension is created between competing survival needs: the need to arouse and maintain awareness of the traumatic process of which we are a part, and the need to forget or deny its existence. In his 1986 Nobel Lecture, Elie Wiesel presented the dilemma in this way: he said, "How could we go on with our daily lives, if we remained constantly aware of the dangers and ghosts surrounding us? The Talmud tells us that without the ability to forget, man would soon cease to learn. Without the ability to forget, man would live in a permanent, paralyzing fear of death."

The need to forget past injuries and to smother present dangers with silence presents a powerful force against which witnesses to past and present wounds must struggle. The siren call of surrender to dangers that seem overpowering can entice an anxious and weary person—even a society as a whole—to embrace the sleep of denial. Like the hypothermic mountaineer who wishes to lie down and rest in the frozen bed of ice and snow—yet knows that she must not succumb to such a suicidal temptation—it is imperative to resist the seductive call to close one's eyes.

Instead, the presence of life-threatening danger requires us, as individuals and human societies, to reach deep within ourselves to find the strength to resist surrender to our losses and our grief. Individuals must join with each other to search for an understanding of how we, as the society of humans, have come to be in such danger, how our actions are influencing our environment, how the losses in our environment are influencing us, and what paths will lead us to safety. We would do well to remember Henry Krystal's words: "The beginning of the traumatic process is the surrender to inevitable danger, which if not interrupted may lead to psychogenic death."

Those who publicly point out the signs and symptoms of collective trauma are subject to the full weight of society's resistance to becoming aware of its own vulnerability. There is a cultural imperative, however, to give voice to collective experiences of traumatic injury. The voice of the witness is an essential anchor to both personal and collective truth, and provides continuity and meaning to the structure and integrity of the community.

The person, man or woman, who speaks out to assert collective truth is sometimes known as a "fool." In royal courts, in past times, the fool was often regarded as a trusted servant and counselor to kings. In modern

CHAPTER 9: PIECES COME TOGETHER

cities he or she is often seen sitting on the sidewalk, cup in hand. The fool speaks of common suffering by his own woundedness. He is at once an outcast and a revered wise man; in some communities he is called a shaman. His woundedness makes him a fearful reminder of individual vulnerability, as well as an example of the transforming effects of traumatic experience. He or she is a person who is thought to bear special wisdom by virtue of being able to traverse the barriers between the invisible and visible worlds, the unconscious and the conscious, the spiritual and the material. He is alive to the wisdom of the sensuous world.

The witness, or fool, appears in many forms in our everyday society. She is the artist, the truthsayer, the magician, the comedian, the madman, and the environmentalist. She is every man and woman who dares to reach into his or her own woundedness, see the face of our collective self reflected there, and to give expression to what she sees.

CHAPTER 10

Finding Our Connections

"An unsung land is a dead land."
—BRUCE CHATWIN

It is tempting to think that the present, collective human experience is entirely new and that we must, therefore, create entirely new solutions to the problems that have arisen. However, it is more likely that the answers will come from within our collective wisdom and history—in other words, that they already exist. Just as the individual who faces traumatic injury must reach deeply within to find his or her anchor to meaning and strength in order to endure, so too must human society reach within its collective experience to identify essential meaning, strength, and value that will enable human life to endure.

In addition, solutions may arise from sources that have previously been dismissed or thought improbable. In times of great danger, a person, or a society, must be willing to reach for help from all available sources and be open to receiving assistance—no matter how unusual its origins might be. (A recent report on current medical advances in treating heretofore "untreatable" post-surgical vascular complications has noted that the leech—the animal once used for medicinal purposes but then discarded by "science" as too primitive and ugly to be a source of healing—is quietly making a comeback into mainstream medicine as an invaluable healer.

This lowly creature, it seems, has much to teach physicians and scientists about how to keep blood flowing and how to care for wounds.) There are many partnerships within and between species that can be lifesaving. If life is to endure, fear, prejudice, and ignorance cannot be permitted to hold sway.

Transmitting Wisdom

The collective wisdom of communities and cultures is passed from one generation to the next in many forms, including legends and myths. The way in which a story is told changes to fit the needs of the present time and place, but the underlying principles and teachings remain essentially the same. Often, stories become so familiar that "the message" they carry is not consciously recognized.

The legend of the Fisher King is one of the earliest incarnations of the legend of the Holy Grail, a story that is now fascinating and familiar to many, just as it was centuries ago. In the 1991 movie *The Fisher King*, the core elements of the legend are lived out in modern terms and in modern times in the hierarchical social and physical world of New York City. In my second encounter with this movie a few years ago, I recognized that it is a quintessential story of traumatic suffering and healing, even though it is presented as a comedy. In fact, the film story is so exact in its graphic detail of the traumatic process that it could serve well as a resource for physicians, psychologists, and other healers to learn the face and facts of traumatic injury. Remarkable also is that a remedy for traumatic loss is provided in this film story, just as it was in the ancient legend.

At the center of the film story of the Fisher King are two heroes who represent opposite trajectories of human response to suffering, which lead, however, to the same psychological and physical state: that of death-in-life. Each man is wounded: one is the victim of violence, the other is an instigator of it. One man searches for meaning to his life in power and

CHAPTER 10: FINDING OUR CONNECTIONS

wealth; the other looks for meaning in his search for the Holy Grail. Each carries a burden of insupportable grief, shame, helplessness, and pain, and is cut off from what he most yearns for.

As the film's story unfolds, the traumatic wounds of the heroes are reflected visually in wounds manifested in the culture (in homelessness, in random violent attacks, in media that thrives on hate, in a dysfunctional medical system) and in the natural environment (geometric slabs of skyscrapers, a chaotic underworld filled with discarded detritus of a gluttonous supraworld). As the heroes lose their connections with all that supports and gives meaning to their lives, both internally and in their social and physical environment, so also does the natural environment appear more sterile and chaotic in extreme forms. It is a wasteland, devoid of the ability to nurture and sustain itself or those who are dependent on it. The people and the environment reflect each other's fragmentation and decay. Their fates are inextricably joined.

Foreshadowed, however, is the remedy, shown in comic, foolish simplicity. The wounded heroes find common ground, literally and figuratively, on a small piece of grassy meadow in Central Park, where they lie naked as children, undefended under the night sky, and tell the stories of who they are and of their quest for meaning. The universe bends to listen to the stories the men tell, and the clouds signal their attentive response. Ultimately, after many detours and much resistance, the two men join in common purpose and compassion, not willingly but because of necessity. Without coming together they cannot survive.

Legends such as the Fisher King and the Holy Grail endure through the centuries because they portray essential problems that confront human existence in every era. The stories also contain collective wisdom, which, if taken to heart, can lead to resolution of conflicts and restoration of health. An essential wisdom of the Fisher King story, in both ancient and new versions, is that connections formed by spontaneous acts of compassion represent the only force strong enough to heal the deep wounds of traumatic destruction and loss. Only by joining together, the story counsels, and bringing the opposite aspects of our selves, our societies, and our natural world into creative connection, can the Grail, or that which represents the primary source of energy and life, be found.

The story of the Grail, encapsulated in this modern visual form, affirms that while the Grail cup itself may be seen as the source of new life, the healing it offers is dependent on the relationship between the wounded person who seeks new life after traumatic collapse and the person who dares to enter into his suffering. Without the compassion of the "other," a person also wounded by life, the cup remains only an inert symbol, out of reach.

Also remarkable in this tale, in both modern and ancient forms, is the assertion that the suffering of wounded human life is transmitted to and expressed in the natural environment. The "wasteland" is the by-product of a human world that has lost its ability to provide a compassionate response to suffering, wherever that suffering is encountered.

A society that forgets or turns its back on the teachings of its legends, the warnings of its fools, and the wisdom of its elders and heroes risks losses that may not be reversible. Nelson Mandela has written about the vital link with nature that sustained him during his years of imprisonment in South Africa. "Some mornings," he wrote, "I walked out into the courtyard and every living thing there, the seagulls and wagtails, the small trees, and even the stray blades of grass seemed to smile and shine in the sun. It was at such times when I perceived the beauty of even this small, closed-in corner of the world, that I knew that someday my people and I would be free." Endurance, the very survival of one's essential integrity, relies on an attunement with "every living thing." In the beauty and smile of a blade of grass, Mandela saw the face of freedom for his people. We must listen and learn from him.

CHAPTER 10: FINDING OUR CONNECTIONS

Who We Are

As she stood on the summit of Denali, having survived two weeks of imprisonment in violent storms and with the safety of home still very far away, Ruth Anne Kocour experienced an acute awareness "of everything past and present and the interconnection of things—that nature is not something outside ourselves, but who we are." As she reflected on the reasons she chose to travel, climb, and struggle in some of the harshest, most challenging environments encountered by humans, she came to the insight that "the value of wild places lies in showing us the way back—that wilderness is but a path back to the center of our souls."

Nature is not outside of us. It is who we are.

To apprehend the inseparability of all life, animate and inanimate, all senses must be attuned. Like the mother in childbirth who can know with her being what all the monitors and doctors cannot—one must learn to listen to the deepest rhythms of one's own life, to hear the life of the invisible and to listen to the lands one walks. The rhythms have been present all along; they were there before we were born; they will remain after we die. Joining with them—joining pulse to pulse, song to song, sorrow to sorrow, strength to strength—this is the task of healing from the wounds of trauma.

"How do we empathize with the Earth when so much is ravaging her?" Terry Tempest Williams asks. In answer she replies:

— *The heartbeats I felt in the womb—two heartbeats, at once, my mother's and my own—are heartbeats of the land. All of life drums and beats, at once, sustaining a rhythm audible only to the spirit. I can drum my heartbeat back into the Earth, beating, hearts beating, my hands on the Earth—like a ruffed grouse, on a log, beating, hearts beating—like a bittern in the marsh, beating, hearts beating. My hands on the Earth beating, hearts beating. I drum back my return.*

We are our mothers and our ancestors; we are the ruffed grouse and the bittern. We are the Earth: not separate. What ravages the Earth ravages us. What injures our mothers, injures us. And what heals the earth will also heal us. The way back to wholeness is through the essential kinship of all things.

The Rhythms of Hope

Songlines, the ancient walking songs of creation, tell the stories of the interconnection of all things. "We are!" say these songs, in walking words and music that have echoed across generations in the cadence of couplets.

Songlines are the stories of creation usually associated with aboriginal communities in Australia. Although there are songlines that are unique to that country and the early people who began life there, songlines by other names exist throughout the world, told in the stories of the first peoples. They are stories of essential identity and of relationships that give structure, texture, and meaning to life.

The writer Bruce Chatwin spent an extended period of time in Australia exploring the history, significance, and meanings of aboriginal songlines. He explains that in the layering, the complexity, and the interweaving of details, songlines provide "a glimpse of a moral universe...in which the structures of kinship reach out to all living men, to all his fellow creatures, and to the rivers, the rocks and the trees."

A songline is not a written document; it is a walking song, remembered and passed down through generations since the beginning of time. The music and words of the songline are not separate from the action of walking the ground, walking the line of creation, that is told in the story of the songline. In the aboriginal tradition it is said that to forget passages, or to sing a couplet of the songline out of order, is to risk undoing creation.

CHAPTER 10: FINDING OUR CONNECTIONS

No less, then, is the damage caused by violating the integrity of the songline by tearing or covering its path: with train tracks or shopping malls, with highways or housing. Such tears, or breaking apart, which disrupt the living story of creation and the moral order manifested in the songline, is a form of traumatic wounding—not only to the history, continuity, and wholeness of a people but also to the interdependence of all created life contained in the songline. Moreover, to break a songline is to take away a principal source of healing: the unity of life. The intuition that something is terribly wrong is based on the observation and accumulating evidence that humanity, as a species, is setting in motion the undoing of creation and along with it the simultaneous undoing of our primary sources of moral order.

Songlines appear in many forms. Like holdfast, which tethers the living kelp plant to the ocean floor, allowing the leaves to stretch up through the water toward the sun, songlines anchor visible created life to its origins deep beneath the surface of the world. These lines of song are invisible, yet known; they mark the path between two worlds: between the unconscious and the conscious, the dream and the waking, the creating and the created. Songlines are the rhythm of hope.

Even the most basic material of an organism, the genome, may be understood as a songline. In the sequence of the genome is given the code unique to life. When one attunes the senses to apprehend the deepest meaning of the code, one can hear music. To some, like Todd Barton and Brent Hugh, the structure of the genome reflects a musical form inherent to life itself. Each of these composers has translated pieces of the structure of life into sound. Hugh describes his musical translation, called "Music of the Genome," as representing that "one small part of that universal harmony that has existed within us for ages, yet has never before been turned into audible music." He further explains that "the beauty and harmony of the universe is the 'real' music and the job of musicians is to tune into some small part of that pre-existing universal harmony and translate it into the more usual type of music, made with human voices and instruments."

Now that these lines of creation have been made visible and audible, it becomes more apparent that attempts to alter or "engineer" such fragile, essential threads of life incur many risks. Greater knowledge of the genome leads also to wonder, as the deep kinship between seemingly dissimilar species is revealed.

There are great strands of many kinds of songlines that have been unrecognized, forgotten, ignored, covered over, or lost to memory. They stretch across all of the earth, giving structure, order, and coherence to life. In them are expressed the beat of the walking body and the waking heart: the urge to live and to create. They lead the way to possibilities of renewal and wholeness. They offer a way back—from grief, from fragmentation and despair, from apocalyptic violence, and from the numbness of life without meaning.

The rhythm of hope is the pulse already there: waiting to be found. The rhythm of the walking song is already known. We have only to put one foot forward, and then the next, to open the senses and to see in each thing we encounter—a rock, a child, a cloud, a honey ant, a father, a fool—the face of woundedness and compassion, a reflection of our own.

Birdwings

*Your grief for what you've lost lifts a mirror
up to where you're bravely working.*

*Expecting the worst, you look, and instead,
here's the joyful face you've been wanting to see.*

*Your hand opens and closes and opens and closes.
If it were always a fist or always stretched open,
you would be paralyzed.*

*Your deepest presence is in every small contracting and expanding,
the two as beautifully balanced and coordinated
as birdwings.*

—RUMI

Notes

Confidentiality is one of the most important elements in building, caring for, and honoring the trust and safety on which helping relationships depend. This obligation is not changed by time, geographic distance, nor whether a person is still living or not. In the course of my work as a counselor and psychotherapist, a researcher, and as a Search and Rescue worker, many have graciously given me their trust. To protect their identity as I write about their experiences, I have altered their names and certain descriptive facts. Their stories remain true. Only where I have received specific permission or the stories I tell are already in the public domain do I knowingly reveal identities.

I have chosen to use the personal pronouns "he" and "she" on the basis of what I think will assist the reader. No bias regarding gender is intended.

Chapter 1. The Search Begins

p 3   "*...that others may live*" is the motto of the National Association for Search and Rescue.

p 12   Lifton's newest book, *Superpower Syndrome: America's Apocalyptic Confrontation with the World* (New York: Nation Books, 2003) builds on his earlier analyses of the disastrous consequences of the misuses of power. His reach is global, but his warnings hit very close to home. Also important to my understanding and formulations developed in this book are Lifton's earlier works, especially *The Broken Connection: On Death and the Continuity of Life* (Arlington, VA: American Psychiatric Press, 1999) and *The Protean Self: Human Resilience in an Age of Fragmentation* (New York: Basic Books, 1993).

NOTES

p 13   The detailed story of Oliver Sacks' accident and recovery is found in his book *A Leg to Stand On* (New York: Simon & Schuster Adult Publishing Group, 1985). His successful effort to convey the full experience of catastrophic personal trauma, from the inside out, is made possible, in part, by the style of his writing. His words match his experience.

p 15   Natan Sharansky discusses his understanding of a spiritual bond with those who have come before him in *Fear No Evil* (New York: Random House, 1988) 360.

p 16   See Gretel Ehrlich, *A Match to the Heart* (New York: Random House, 1994) 83.

Chapter 2. Something Is Terribly Wrong

p 19   "...*something is terribly missing*..."is from David Abram, *The Spell of the Sensuous* (New York: Random House, 1996) 270.

p 20   The Trauma Research Center of Seattle sponsored the pilot study "Maternal Experience of Trauma in Childbirth." Members of the Research team included Hilary Bolles, M.Ed., Monica Bristow, Ph.D., Susan Flagler, R.N, Penny Simkin, O.T.R., and Karen Merriam, M.S.S. (the author). Additional assistance and direction was provided by Myra Kim Faust, O.T.R., Kate Grutz, M.A., Billie Z. Lawson, M.S.W., Kathie McCarthy, M.A., Marianne Pettersen, M.S.W., Barabara Stratton, M.B.A., Brenda Buck, R.D., and Andrea Corage-Baden. At the time our study was initiated (in 1990), our searches of the professional literature yielded no articles related to women's experiences of trauma in childbirth.

Chapter 3. How Connections Are Lost

p 35   "*One looks into the abyss in order to see beyond it.*" is from Robert Jay Lifton's book *Destroying the World to Save It* (New York: Henry Holt and Company, LLC, 1999) 344.

p 37   See Benyakar, M., Kutz, I., Dasberg, H., and Stern, M. J. "The collapse of a structure: a structural approach to trauma." *Journal of Traumatic Stress* (1989) 2:431–462.

p 39   Joe Simpson's account of his terrifying experiences on Siula Grande are recorded in his book *Touching the Void* (New York: HarperCollins, 1988) and in the documentary movie *Touching the Void,* A Film by Kevin Macdonald. DVD Video: MGM Home Entertainment, IFC Films, 2003.

p 43   "*The cold was taking me again...*"from Simpson, *Touching the Void* (158–159).

p 44   "*I lost something then. I lost—me.*" From the DVD Video, *Touching the Void*. See also the DVD Video Featurettes "Making of *Touching the Void*," "Return to Siula Grande," and "What Happened Next" for accounts of the direct effects of making the movie on all involved in the project. In these documentary scenes and interviews, the viewer is able to see the fragmenting aspects of trauma as they happen. Social and working relationships on location fracture, and Joe Simpson is re-traumatized, as an unexpected and unintended consequence of the filming.

p 45   Gretel Ehrlich refers frequently to the "gap" or "bardo state" in *A Match to the Heart* (40–41). Her understanding of this "state between life and death" derives from her reading of the *Tibetan Book of the Dead*, as translated by Chogyan Trungpa Rinpoche.

p 46   See Ruth Anne Kocour, as told to Michael Hodgson, *Facing the Extreme* (New York: St. Martin's Press, 1998) 195.

p 47   See Sacks, *A Leg to Stand On* (63, 86, 158–159).

p 47   For a fuller discussion of this quotation from Primo Levi, see Jerome Groopman, *The Measure of Our Days: New Beginnings at Life's End* (New York: The Penguin Group, 1997) 56. Also see Primo Levi, *The Drowned and the Saved* (New York: Simon & Schuster, Inc., 1986).

p 47   Henry Krystal's writings on trauma are pivotal to the development of an understanding of the traumatic process. See Henry Krystal, "Trauma and affects." *The Psychoanalytic Study of the Child* (1978) 33:81–116.

p 48   *The Pawnbroker*. A Lions Gate Film. Landau Company. Directed by Sidney Lumet. Based on the novel by E. L. Wallant. 1964.

p 48   *The Fisher King*. Produced by Debra Hill and Lynda Obst. Directed by Terry Gilliam. Written by Richard LaGravenese. TRISTAR Videocassette. 1991.

p 51   "May" is the name I have given to a counselor with the Bereavement Program of Hospice Partners of the Central Coast. The story is true in all of its details except for the names.

Chapter 4. Energies to Survive

p 53   "Survival is as much a matter of grace as fight." See Ehrlich, *A Match to the Heart* (134).

p 54   See Ehrlich, *A Match to the Heart* (134, 124–125).

p 54   See Joseph Campbell, *The Power of Myth*, with Bill Moyers. (New York: Doubleday, 1988) 217–218. The T. S. Eliot quotation is cited from this same source (217).

p 57   Aron Ralston's book, *Between a Rock and a Hard Place* (New York: Atria Books, 2004), provides another intimate glimpse into the heart of traumatic experience. His account draws on his journal entries as well as his videotapes of his ordeal. See also Aron Ralston's article "Trapped" in *Outside* (September, 2004):52–60, 115–116.

p 59   See Beck Weathers. With Stephen G. Michaud. *Left for Dead: My Journey Home from Everest*. (New York: Random House, Inc., 2000) 59–61, 8, 63–64.

p 60   See Antoine de Saint-Exupéry, "Prisoners of Sand," in *Wind, Sand and Stars*, translated by Lewis Galantiére (San Diego: Harcourt, Inc., 1939, 1967) 146–147, 159.

NOTES

p 62 Oliver Sacks has written extensively about the relationship of music to neuropsychological functioning. In this instance he is able to draw on his own experience to document the central organizing function of music, which takes on a metaphysical role in his recovery from traumatic injury. See Sacks, *A Leg to Stand On* (13, 116, 120–122).

p 65 See Art Davidson, "Minus 148°: The Winter Ascent of Mt. McKinley" in *Courage & Misfortune*. (Seattle: Mountaineers Books, Anthology Series Vol. II, 2001) 219.

p 66 See Natan Sharansky, *Fear No Evil* (New York: Random House, 1988) 374–375.

p 66 Jerome Groopman addresses the subject of hope from the perspective of the intricate neurochemical and psychobiological responses to illness, traumatic injury, and grief. Hope, he explains, is not a simple matter of mind over body, or of individual will, but rather a complex mix of personal, social, physical, and spiritual attitudes and activities. See Jerome Groopman, *The Anatomy of Hope: How People Prevail in the Face of Illness* (New York: Random House, 2004).

Chapter 5. Principles, Plans, and Strategies

p 69 *"Believe in your own heart...."* See Sharansky, *Fear No Evil* (375).

p 71 See Sharansky, *Fear No Evil* (375).

p 72 See Sharansky, *Fear No Evil* (8, 20, 28).

p 74 See Nelson Mandela, *Long Walk to Freedom: The Autobiography of Nelson Mandela* (Boston: Little, Brown & Company, 1994) 340.

p 76 See Mandela, *Long Walk to Freedom* (341).

Chapter 6. Legacies: Transmission of Trauma

p 81 *"Perhaps we are like stones..."* from Susan Griffin, *A Chorus of Stones* (New York: Doubleday, 1992) 8.

p 86 See Lenore Terr, M.D., *Too Scared to Cry: Psychic Trauma in Childhood* (New York: Harper & Row Publishers, 1990). In this book, and in many journal articles, Terr documents the difficulties experienced over time of the children and families affected by the Chowchilla bus kidnapping. One of her great contributions to understanding the effects of childhood traumatic experience is her documentation of the longevity and severity of symptoms, as illustrated by their appearance in popular literature and films whose creators were traumatized as children.

p 89 See Elie Wiesel, Nobel Lecture, "Hope, Despair and Memory," December 11, 1986.

p 91 See Elie Wiesel, *All Rivers Run to the Sea: Memoirs* (New York: Alfred A. Knopf, Inc, 1995) 339.

p 92 See Maya Angelou, *I Know Why the Caged Bird Sings* (New York: Random House, 1969) 71–73.

p 94 See Alf Bøe, *Edvard Munch*, translated from the Norwegian by Robert Ferguson (Barcelona: Ediciones Poligrafia, SA, 1989) 20.

Chapter 7. Legacies: The Brain, the Will, and the Body

p 97 "There was a lesion…" is from Sacks, *A Leg to Stand On* (46).

p 98 See Terr, *Too Scared to Cry* (120–145).

p 107 See Sacks, *A Leg to Stand On* (43, 46, 48).

p 108 *The Pawnbroker*. A Lions Gate Film. Landau Company. Directed by Sidney Lumet. Based on the novel by E. L. Wallant. 1964.

Chapter 8. Finding the Face of Compassion

p 111 "The best we can do…" See Campbell, *The Power of Myth* (197).

p 111 See Ehrlich, *A Match to the Heart* (22, 85–89, 91).

p 113 I am reminded by these words "It doesn't fit" of the familiar passage from Shakespeare's *Hamlet*, "The time is out of joint" (Act 1, Scene 5). Certain losses, such as the murder of a daughter-in-law and her unborn child or of a father, can disrupt one's basic orientation, and the event may be seen as evidence of a world order gone awry.

p 115 For a useful discussion of the psychophysiological imperatives for safety in the work of trauma treatment, see Babette Rothschild, *The Body Remembers: The Psychophysiology of Trauma and Trauma Treatment* (New York: W.W. Norton & Company, Inc., 2000).

p 120 See Jon Krakauer, *Into Thin Air: A Personal Account of the Mount Everest Disaster* (New York: Random House, 1997). Krakauer was one of the climbers in camp with Weathers and recounts his and the other climbers' reactions to the unfolding traumatic events.

p 121 Beck Weathers' autobiographical book detailing his experiences on Everest is enriched by inclusion of commentary and reflections by his wife Peach. See Weathers, *Left for Dead* (64–65, 68–69).

p 121 See Joe Simpson, *Dark Shadows Falling* (London: Jonathan Cape, Random House, 1996) 205.

p 122 See Bernard Lown, M.D., *The Lost Art of Healing* (New York: Ballantine Books, 1999) 286.

p 122 See Groopman, *The Measure of Our Days* (90–91).

NOTES

p 125 *"Solvitur ambulando"* is the title of Chapter 5 in Oliver Sacks' book *A Leg to Stand On* and also expresses a central theme in Bruce Chatwin's book *The Songlines*.

p 126 See Antoine de Saint-Exupéry, "Prisoners of Sand," *Wind, Sand and Stars*. (Harcourt, Inc, 1939) 170–173.

Chapter 9. Pieces Come Together

p 127 *"Nature is not only…"* from Edvard Munch. See Internet, <www.artquotes.net/masters/munch-edvard-quotes.htm>.

p 131 For a thorough discussion of the human loss of connection with the sensual world, see Abram, *The Spell of the Sensuous*.

p 135 See Lown, *The Lost Art of Healing* (47).

p 137 See Terry Tempest Williams, *Refuge: An Unnatural History of Family and Place* (New York: Random House, 1991) 288.

p 139 See Robert Jay Lifton, *Destroying the World to Save It: Aum Shinrikyō, Apocalyptic Violence, and the New Global Terrorism* (New York: Metropolitan Books, 1999) 4–5.

p 140 See Lawrence Wright, "The Kingdom of Silence" in *The New Yorker* (January 5, 2004): 48–73.

p 140 See Ron Powers, "The Apocalypse of Adolescence" in *The Atlantic Monthly* (March, 2002): 58–74.

p 143 See "Truthsayer" at Wikipedia: Truthsayer is a fictional profession in the Dune universe created by Frank Herbert. A truthsayer is a trained individual who is able to detect whether someone is lying by observing their body language. In the Dune universe, truthsayers are used widely in politics and trade. <http://en.wikipedia.org/wiki/Truthsayer>. October 29, 2005.

Chapter 10. Finding Our Connections

p 145 *"An unsung land…"* from Bruce Chatwin, *The Songlines* (New York: Penguin Books, 1988) 52.

p 148 See Mandela, *Long Walk to Freedom* (441).

p 149 See Kocour, *Facing the Extreme* (233–234).

p 149 See Williams, *Refuge* (282–283).

p 150 See Chatwin, *The Songlines* (70, 72–73).

p 151 See Todd Barton, "Genome Music: Music derived from dna code." MP3.com. <http//www.mp3.com/metaScape, and http//www.mind.net/music/genome/gen2.htm>. 2001, liner notes.

p 151 See Brent Hugh, "Music of the Genome" on the Internet at <brenthugh.com>.

— 159 —

References

Books

Abram, David. *The Spell of the Sensuous*. New York: Random House, 1996.

Angelou, Maya. *I Know Why the Caged Bird Sings*. New York: Random House, 1969.

Campbell, Joseph. With Bill Moyers. *The Power of Myth*. New York: Doubleday, 1988.

Chatwin, Bruce. *The Songlines*. New York: The Penguin Group, 1987.

Davidson, Art. "Minus 148°: The Winter Ascent of Mt. McKinley" in *Courage & Misfortune*. The Mountaineers Anthology Series, Vol. II. Seattle: The Mountaineers Books, 2001.

Ehrlich, Gretel. *A Match to the Heart*. New York: Random House, Inc., 1994.

Griffin, Susan. *A Chorus of Stones*. New York: Doubleday, 1992.

Groopman, Jerome M.D. *The Anatomy of Hope: How People Prevail in the Face of Illness*. New York: Random House, Inc., 2004.

Groopman, Jerome M.D. *The Measure of Our Days: New Beginnings at Life's End*. New York: The Penguin Group, 1997.

Kocour, Ruth Anne. *Facing the Extreme* (as told to Michael Hodgson). New York: St. Martin's Press, 1998.

Krakauer, Jon. *Into Thin Air: A Personal Account of the Mount Everest Disaster*. New York: Random House, 1997.

LaGravenese, Richard. *The Fisher King: The Book of the Film*. New York: Applause Theatre Book Publishers, 1991.

Levi, Primo. *The Drowned and the Saved*. New York: Simon & Schuster, Inc, 1986.

Lifton, Robert Jay. *The Broken Connection: On Death and the Continuity of Life*. Arlington, VA: American Psychiatric Press, 1979.

Lifton, Robert Jay. *Destroying the World to Save It: Aum Shinrikyō, Apocalyptic Violence, and the New Global Terrorism*. New York: Henry Holt and Company, LLC, 1999.

REFERENCES

Lifton, Robert Jay. *The Protean Self: Human Resilience in an Age of Fragmentation.* New York: Basic Books, 1993.

Lifton, Robert Jay. *Superpower Syndrome: Americas's Apocalyptic Confrontation with the World.* Thunder Mouth Press: Nation Books, 2003.

Lown, Bernard, M.D. *The Lost Art of Healing.* New York: Ballantine Books, 1996.

Mandela, Nelson. *Long Walk to Freedom: The Autobiography of Nelson Mandela.* Boston: Little, Brown & Company, 1994.

NiCarthy, Ginny, Merriam, Karen, and Coffman, Sandra. *Talking It Out: A Guide to Groups for Abused Women.* Seattle: Seal Press, 1984.

Ralston, Aron. *Between a Rock and a Hard Place.* New York: Atria Books, 2004.

Rothschild, Babette. *The Body Remembers: The Psychophysiology of Trauma and Trauma Treatment.* New York: W.W. Norton & Company, Inc, 2000.

Rumi. *The Essential Rumi.* Translations by Coleman Barks with John Moyne. New York: HarperCollins Publishers, 1996.

Sacks, Oliver. *Awakenings.* New York: Random House, 1973.

Sacks, Oliver. *A Leg to Stand On.* New York: Simon & Schuster Adult Publishing Group, 1985.

Saint-Exupéry, Antoine de. *Wind, Sand and Stars.* Harcourt, Inc, 1939.

Sharansky, Natan. *Fear No Evil.* New York: Random House, Inc., 1988.

Simpson, Joe. *Dark Shadows Falling.* London: Jonathan Cape, Random House, 1997.

Simpson, Joe. *Touching the Void.* New York: HarperCollins Publishers, Inc., 1988.

Terr, Lenore. *Too Scared to Cry: Psychic Trauma in Childhood.* New York: Harper & Row Publishers, 1990.

van der Kolk, B. A., McFarlane, A. C. and Weisaeth. L. (Eds.). *Traumatic Stress: The Effects of Overwhelming Experience on Mind, Body and Society.* New York: The Guilford Press, 1996.

Wagoner, David. "Lost" in *Traveling Light: Collected and New Poems.* University of Illinois Press, 1999.

Wallant, E. L. *The Pawnbroker.* New York: Harcourt, Brace & World, 1961.

Weathers, Beck. With Stephen G. Michaud. *Left for Dead: My Journey Home from Everest.* New York: Random House, Inc., 2000.

Wiesel, Elie. *Memoirs: All Rivers Run to the Sea.* New York: Alfred A. Knopf, 1995.

Williams, Terry Tempest. *Refuge: An Unnatural History of Family and Place.* New York: Random House, 1991.

Film, Videotape & DVD

The Fisher King. Produced by Debra Hill and Lynda Obst. Directed by Terry Gilliam. Written by Richard LaGravenese. 137 min. TRISTAR. 1991. Videocassette.

The Pawnbroker. Lions Gate. Landau Company. Directed by Sidney Lumet. Based on the novel by E. L. Wallant. 1964.

Touching the Void. A Film by Kevin Macdonald. MGM Home Entertainment. 2004.

Journal Articles

Benyakar, M., Kutz, I., Dasberg, H. and Stern, M. J. "The collapse of a structure: a structural approach to trauma," *Journal of Traumatic Stress* (1989) 2:431–462.

Krystal, H. "Trauma and affects," *The Psychoanalytic Study of the Child* (1978) 33:81–116.

Terr, L. "Children of Chowchilla: A Study of Psychic Trauma," *Psychoanalytic Study of the Child* (1979) 34: 547–623.

Terr, L. "Time and Trauma." *Psychoanalytic Study of the Child* (1984) 39:633–665.

Other Publications

Lown, Bernard, M.D. "Never Whisper in the Presence of Wrong." Excerpts from addresses to Meetings of International Physicians for the Prevention of Nuclear War. 1985–1993. <http://www.ippnw.org/NeverWhisper.html>.

Munch, Edvard. <http://www.artquotes.net/masters/munch-edvard-quotes.htm>.

Powers, Ron. "The Apocalypse of Adolescence," in *The Atlantic Monthly* (March, 2002): 58–74.

Ralston, Aron. "Trapped," in *Outside* (September, 2004): 52–60, 115–116.

Wiesel, Elie. Interview. June 29, 1996, Sun Valley, Idaho. <http://www.achievement.org>. Copyright 2002 American Academy of Achievement.

Wright, Lawrence. "The Kingdom of Silence," in *The New Yorker* (January 5, 2004): 48–73.

Music

Barton, Todd. "Genome Music: Music derived from dna code." MP3.com. <http://www.mp3.com/metaScape, and http//www.mind.net/music/genome/gen2.htm>. 2001.

Hugh, Brent. "Music of the Genome." <http://www.brenthugh.com>.

Index

Abram, David, 19, 159
alexithymia, 102–104
alienation, 32–34
Anatomy of Hope, 66–67
Angelou, Maya, 14, 92–93
apocalypse, 137
   nihilism and, 140
   visions of, 138–139
Asahara, Shoko, 139, 141
Aum Shinrikyō, 139
Auschwitz, 70
authentic self, 71, 78
Ayers, A. Jean, 123

Barton, Todd, 151
Benyakar, Mordechai, 37–38
Bible:
   book of Psalms, 72
   crucifixion in, 44–45
bin Laden, Osama, 139–141
"Birdwings," 153
Blue John Canyon, 57
Bonington, Chris, 77
Braniff, Blaine, 111, 115
Burleson, Todd, 120

Campbell, Joseph, 54, 71, 111
Chatwin, Bruce, 145, 150, 159
childbirth:
   death thoughts and, 49

   expectations of, 81–82
   experiences, 21–22, 81, 87
   invalidation in, 26
   isolation in, 92
   subjective appraisal of, 33, 149
   trauma research, viii, 20, 23, 28
Chillon:
   Castle/Chateau of, 84
   Prisoner of Chillon, 84
Chowchilla, CA:
   kidnapping, 87, 95, 98
cognitive constriction, 104–105
compassion, 18, 91, 95, 111, 127–128
   failures of, 117–119
   fatigue, 118
   necessity of, 148
connections:
   effects of trauma on, 20, 97
   finding, 145–162
   human and ecological, 18, 127, 132–136, 149
   in stories, 55, 93
   inner voice, 55
   interconnection of human souls, 15, 18
   loss of, 35–52, 135
   necessity of, 17–18
   reverse, 15, 56
   support for, 20
connective tissue, 36–37
contagion effect, 86

danger, 18–20, 26–27, 38–39, 115–116
   hope and, 65
   overwhelming, 15
   psychological, 28–30
   resisting, 63
   responses to, 97–99, 153
   suicide and, 49
   surrender to, 42, 47–48, 67, 83, 116, 139, 141–142
Davidson, Art, 64–65
death:
   attitudes toward, 38, 44, 79, 119–122, 130
   death-in-life, 45–46, 48, 77, 146
   fear of, 121
   hypothermia and, 38, 41
   near-death, 28, 60, 112
   psychogenic, 47, 141–142
   resistance to, 41, 59
   suicide and, 49, 139
   surrender to, 63
Denali, 45, 64, 149
Destroying the World to Save It, 12
Dickinson, Emily, 28
dignity, 66, 70, 74–76
dread, 46, 54, 66, 82–83, 115
   danger and, 25–27, 30, 140
   denial and, 138
   expectation and, 85
   foreboding and, 17, 19
   legacies of, 85, 129–130
   overcoming, 63, 66, 119
   resistance to, 41
   suffering and, 12–13, 97
   transmitting, 87, 137

Ehrlich, Gretel, 16, 45, 53–54, 62, 111–112, 124–125
Eliot, T. S., 54
endurance, 14, 59, 70, 74, 77–78, 127, 148
Everest, Mount, 58–59, 76, 105, 119–121

extinction, 13, 38, 131–132, 138

Facing the Extreme, 14
faith, 41, 64–65, 72
Fear No Evil, 15, 71–73
Fisher King, 48–49, 146–147
flashback, 25, 48
fragmentation, 17, 34, 78, 97
   healing and, 125
   human and environmental, 147
   self, 109
   will power and, 106

genome, 151
grace, 24, 53–54, 61–62, 78, 112
Grail:
   legend and symbol, 54, 146–148
Great Depression, 91
grief, 25, 101
   environment and, 131–133, 136–137
   healing, 79, 142, 152–153
   motivator, 60
   physical injury and, 31
   somatic expression of, 84
   traumatic, 50–52, 108–109, 112–114
Griffin, Susan, vii, 81
Groopman, Jerome, 66–67, 122

Hamlet, 15, 158
healer, 112, 114, 127
   broken contract, 135
   honesty of, 116
   strengths, 33, 122–123
   suffering and, 114
   wounded, 119
healing, 18, 30, 34, 145, 149
   compassion and, 118
   reciprocal relationship in, 111, 148
   safety and, 115
   source of, 151
   stories of, 146
holistic medicine, 118

INDEX

Holocaust, 12–13, 47, 88–89, 91, 108
hope:
    apocalypse and, 138–140
    false hope, 64–66
    holding for another, 68
    resilience and, 67
    rhythm of, 151–152
    safety and, 116
    suicide and, 49
    youth and, 140
    Zaziwe, 76
Hospice, vii, 51
Hugh, Brent, 151
hypervigilance, 97, 98
    as communication, 99, 100
    as safety, 101
hypothermia, 38–39, 41–42, 58, 63, 76, 105

I Know Why the Caged Bird Sings, 92

Jesus, last words of, 44–45

Kocour, Ruth Anne, 14, 45–46, 149
Krystal, Henry, 47, 142

Left for Dead, 58–59
Leg to Stand On, 13, 34
Levi, Primo, 47, 156
Lifton, Robert Jay, 12, 35, 43, 139–140, 154
Long Walk to Freedom, 74–76
Lord Byron, Gordon George, 84
"Lost," 1
Lost Art of Healing, 14
Lown, Bernard, 14, 121, 134–135, 137
Luria, A. R., 32–33

malingering, 107
Mandela, Nelson, 74–76, 78, 148
Match to the Heart, 54
medical industrial complex, 135

memory:
    breakdown of, 108
    buried, 9–10, 78, 84, 91, 108
    genetic, 125
    lost, 46–47, 136, 140, 152
    recovering, 103–104, 106, 110
    silence and, 91
    somatic/body, 61, 124
    traumatic, 22, 79, 136
miracle, 53, 58, 66, 69, 126
modulation, 37, 123–124
Munch, Edvard, 94–95, 127
music:
    as expression of trauma, 12, 93, 95
    genome, 151–152
    survival and, 61–63, 78, 157
    walking and, 125, 150

Namba, Yasuko, 119
National Association for Search and Rescue, 3
Nazerman, Sol, 48, 108, 141
nightmares, 83

pain, 22–23, 28, 44, 82–83, 85, 114, 133, 141
Pawnbroker, 48, 108, 141
Powers, Ron, 140

radioactive fallout, 136–137
Ralston, Aron, 57–58, 63, 78
Refuge, 13
Rumi, 153

Sacks, Oliver, 13, 30–34, 46–47, 49, 61–63, 97, 107–109, 117, 124
safety, 85, 99–100, 115–116, 130
Saint-Exupéry, Antoine de, 14, 60, 125–126
Science, 135
Scream, 94
Search and Rescue, 3

search dog, 3–8, 16
Second World War, 88
self-regulation, 38, 73, 79, 101
Sensory Integration, 123–124
Seven Sisters, 133
Sharansky, Avital, 72–73
Sharansky, Natan, 15, 55–56, 65–66, 69, 71–73, 76, 138–139
silence, 21, 83
   as communication, 12, 86, 91–92, 114
   as protection, 86, 93, 142
   at the center of trauma, 26, 32, 44, 51
   breaking, 85, 89, 137–138
   in the environment, 134
   shared, 88, 115–116
Simpson, Joe, 13, 39–43, 49, 56–57, 62–63, 67–68, 77–78, 82, 121
Siula Grande, 39, 56–57, 62, 77
songlines, 150–152
structural collapse, 37, 138
suicide, 49
   apocalypse and, 138–141
survival, 10, 17, 30, 39, 42, 53, 63, 65–66, 74, 105, 119, 141, 148,

Terr, Lenore, 86–87, 98
terror, 13, 18, 21–22, 31, 75, 79, 83, 94–95, 97, 101, 106, 123, 129–130, 137, 138
   speechless, 102
terrorism, 12, 133, 140
This Game of Ghosts, 14
Touching the Void, 14, 39, 77
trauma:
   aloneness, 44–45, 109
   awareness of, 141
   bardo, gap, hiatus, hole, 33, 45–46, 49, 54, 115, 156
   depiction of, 84, 146
   early stages of, 19–20, 47, 116
   environmental, 18, 94, 131, 133–134, 148

   experience of, 13, 20, 117
   process of, 13, 21, 26, 35–40, 64, 132, 139, 156
   resolution of, 79
   return of, 85, 119
   suicide and, 139
   systemic, 37
   transmission of, 85, 87–88, 93–94

validation, 30, 33–34, 124–125, 130
   lack of, 26, 29, 30, 33–34, 117, 136
Volans, Kevin, 62

Wagoner, David, 1
walking, 124–125
   rhythm of, 128, 152
   songs, 150
wasteland, 18, 134, 138–139, 147–148
   heroes of, 141
   internal, 138
   suicide and, 139
Weathers, Beck, 58–59, 76–77, 119–121
Weathers, Peach, 120–121
Wiesel, Elie, 12, 88–89, 91, 141–142
Williams, Terry Tempest, 13, 136–137, 149
willpower, 106–110
Wind, Sand and Stars, 14, 125–126
   "Prisoners of the Sand," 60
wisdom, 143, 148
   collective, 145–147
   transmitting, 146
witness, 18, 57, 112, 143
   need for, 67, 77, 122, 127–128
   survivors as, 89
witnessing:
   affirmation in, 9, 113–114
   collaboration in, 116, 128, 137
   discomfort in, 94, 118, 120–121
   imperative for, 12, 141–142

Yates, Simon, 39–40, 43, 56–57, 67–68, 78

Give the Gift of
SEARCHING FOR CONNECTION

An Exploration of Trauma, Culture, and Hope

to Your Friends and Colleagues

GO TO **www.searchingforconnection.com**

CHECK YOUR LEADING BOOKSTORE
OR ORDER HERE

❏ **YES**, I want _____ copies of *Searching for Connection* at $22.95 each, plus $4.95 shipping per book (California residents please add $1.66 sales tax per book). All orders must be paid in U.S. funds. Allow 15 days for delivery.

My check or money order for $_____ is enclosed.

Please charge my: ❏ Visa   ❏ MasterCard
                    ❏ Discover   ❏ American Express

Name _____

Organization _____

Address _____

City/State/Zip _____

Phone_____ Email _____

Card # _____

Exp. Date_____ Signature _____

Please make your check payable and return to:

Truthsayer Press
P.O. Box 1244 • San Luis Obispo, CA 93406

Call your credit card order to: (800) 326-9001
Fax: (805) 541-1360